WHO TRAINS, WINS
Matthew Black

How anyone can train for SUCCESS & WEALTH with the MARTIAL ARTS

Train and Grow Rich

MATTHEW BLACK

WHO TRAINS, WINS
© 2025 First Edition, Matthew Black
ISBN # 979-8-9942332-3-8
Published by FWS Investments
WhoTrainsWins@proton.me
WhoTrainsWins.com

All rights reserved.
Registered and copyrighted. No portion of this book may be reproduced in any form without written permission from the publisher or author, except as permitted by copyright law.

This publication is designed to provide accurate and authoritative information in regard to the subject matter covered. It is sold with the understanding that neither the author nor the publisher is engaged in rendering legal, health, medical or other professional services. The opinions and ideas contained in this book are not to be used as a replacement to individual medical assessments and personalized health regimes. The training methods, exercises, nutritional guidance, and physical activities described in this book carry inherent risk of injury. The author and publisher expressly disclaim any liability for any injury, loss, or damage incurred as a direct or indirect result of the use or application of any content in this book. Readers are advised to consult a qualified medical professional before beginning any exercise, training, or dietary program.

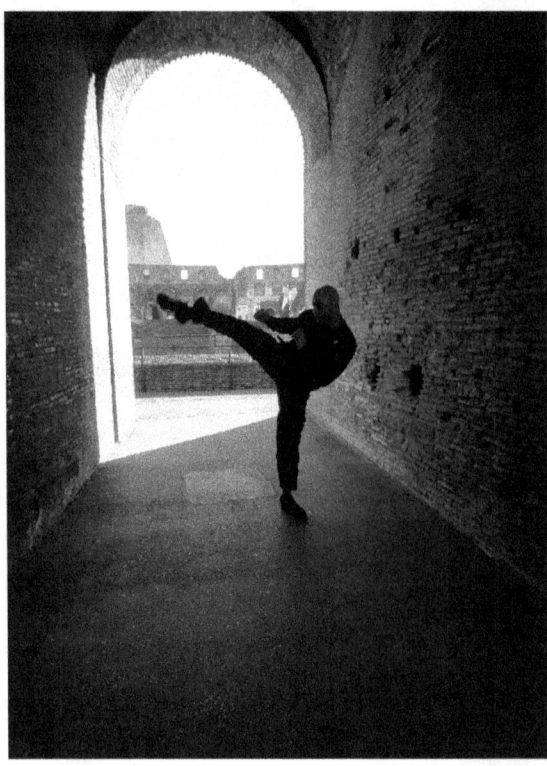

Contents

Contents   3
Preface   4
Introduction   5
Chapter 1 – SEEK DISCIPLINE   6
Chapter 2 – EMBRACE a STYLE   18
Chapter 3 – MANIFEST your WARRIOR   35
Chapter 4 – MASTER EMOTIONS   49
Chapter 5 – FIGHT FEAR   65
Chapter 6 – EMBODY RESPECT   76
Chapter 7 – HONE the PHYSICAL   91
Chapter 8 – FUEL the VESSEL   107
Chapter 9 – TIMING RECOVERY   134
Chapter 10 – SHARPEN the MIND   143
Chapter 11 – SPIRITUAL ACTIVATION   159
Chapter 12 – FLOW in ZEN   179
Chapter 13 – THE MARTIAL TAO   192
Chapter 14 – TEACH to LEARN   209
Chapter 15 – PURIFY the WARRIOR   220
Chapter 16 – SUCCESS BREEDS SUCCESS   234
Appendix   248
Acknowledgments   251
Bibliography   252

Preface

> *"Know your outcome and you don't worry about the journey."*—Unknown

"Who Trains, Wins." is the study of the benefits of martial arts training, and how I translated and applied those lessons for success in every aspect of my life. This tome is an aggregation of wisdom from instructors, combatants, and peers. This project started as the recording of my daily training, progress and schedule. It has evolved over the last 20 years into the translation of the lessons, poignant moments and the motivational ideas that encouraged me throughout training and doing.

My university education was in criminal law, and psychology. I am a security contractor, investigator, K9 handler, pilot, motorcyclist, and now author, but first and foremost, I am a martial artist.

I earned a black belt in Tae Kwon Do, and hold ranked belts in Shaolin Gong-fu, BJJ, and Shotokan Karate. While traveling to over 30 countries, I sought training with Masters of martial styles from Budo in Japan, Kushti in India, Arnis with Guru Dan Inosanto to Krav Maga, boxing and Muay Thai. Over the years I continued developing in the martial way with sky marshal, paramilitary & counter terrorism training, and took specialized contracts operating as a K9 handler and a high risk close protection operative.

Writing this book has proven to be a multi-year catharsis. It is my current stage in learning how to teach. I have much more to learn. In writing this book I reinforced that I must continue in my own training, in eating well, in meditating, just as I have advised here. Following the martial way provided a comprehensive operational system that led me to many of life's successes. I hope this chronicle will assist others with their journey.

I wish you health, wealth and success,

Matthew Black

Introduction

Welcome to an examination into the foundations of a complete martial artist, and how their application translates into a successful life for the practitioner. It is not a book of techniques and movements or which style is better. It is a book that encourages the exploration of your inner warrior and everything required to make the most of your personal development. Just like in a physical fight, the greater degree of the interaction is mental, and an internal struggle. Broader success is the result of laser focus, honed skills, and goals made and achieved. The only barrier to repeatable victory is effort. It is as simple as practicing to make your autonomic actions and reactions regimented and predictable in any environment, hostile or not.

The martial arts teach us dedication, work ethic, respect for others and cooperation to bring you to a higher level of performance. The tools you gain are invaluable for yourself and multiplied when you share them with those around you.

When you train with others, you help them to experiment and improve. You both get to face live action stress stimulus in which to practice and gain invaluable feedback from. There is also the bonus of learning how to operate as an individual inside of a historied entity.

Who Trains, Wins, has been crafted to encompass the human experience and it is addressed to the individual who fervently wants to become the optimal version of themselves. Growing rich in all facets of life is the result of applying martial discipline and focused effort to every challenge you face from today forward. The best time to start training to win was yesterday, the next best time is today.

CHAPTER 1 – SEEK DISCIPLINE

"Without discipline, success is impossible."
Chuck Norris, 1987

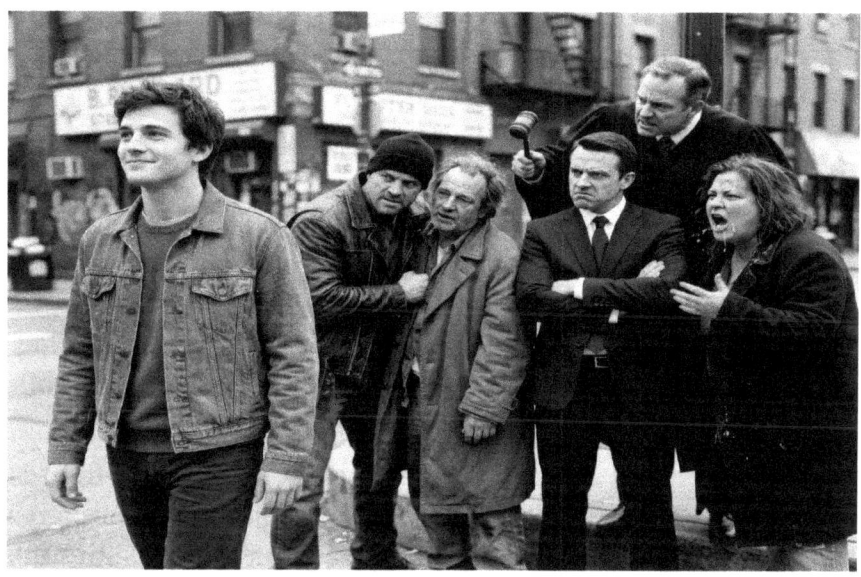

There's a Fight Coming

If there is one certainty to this life, it is that a fight is coming your way, and soon. Not maybe. Not just if you're unlucky. Guaranteed.

The threat of an impending struggle should excite you to your core. You should relish the chance to prove your worth and test your capability. Victory or defeat, either way you will learn and grow.

A fight is coming? Good.

Thinking back, I remember my first physical altercation in the first grade, just before school started at 0800. Standing in line for class, an argument over what order the line was supposed to be started. In quick escalation, I was in a hands–on struggle, one I had no preparation for, ending in a head–lock administered to me by another student. Even though the teachers broke it up quickly, it was clear that I had a very big hole in my life skills that needed filling, and right away. Soon after, I learned about Bruce Lee and self–defense with the Martial Arts, thus my journey had begun.

This cute little schoolyard tussle was an early test. It bore a valuable lesson at a cheap price, because no one got hurt. Every test is a rare opportunity for you to shine. Remember — diamonds are made under heat and pressure. The struggles you face aren't obstacles to avoid; they're the forge that transforms you into something harder, clearer, more valuable. They definitely clear up any misconceptions and illusory capabilities. Real world experience is a quick instructor.

Let's be crystal clear: showing up unprepared for a fight is not bravery. It's stupidity. The wise warrior actively prepares for the battles ahead. The disciplined fighter trains before the fight arrives, not after. I will emphasize, your responsibility to be ready for the fight never ends.

Martial arts training is more than conditioning. It is a philosophy of readiness, a commitment to constant improvement, a lifestyle built on the foundation of discipline.

The mark of a developed, mature human is self–discipline. But what is discipline?

It's not about being harsh with yourself. It's not about punishment or rigid inflexibility. Discipline is a learned behavior displayed through daily diligence in performing your chosen habits and actions.

Personal discipline can be experienced in your life immediately by setting a goal and then doing whatever it takes to accomplish it. In martial arts, discipline reveals itself in the journey of a black belt—who is simply a white belt that never quit. Every day from the moment they began, the black belt chose to continue training, to submit to testing, to show up when it was hard.

For this reason, people across the world respect martial artists. They have proven their discipline. The process of becoming a martial artist fundamentally changes the person who commits to and achieves mastery. The discipline of the martial artist's lifestyle becomes obvious as everyone around recognizes the sacrifice and overall improvement of character that the practitioner reveals.

When your peers and teachers recognize your progress—through graduation to a new rank, participation in tournaments, a successful defense on the street—the hard work, dedication, and discipline manifest and garner the respect they deserve.

You might ask: can't any difficult pursuit build discipline? Why martial arts specifically?

The answer lies in how martial arts training rewires your brain and body simultaneously.

Neuroplasticity

Scientists can actually see the changes happening in your brain. Let me explain what they've discovered. Research on elite karate athletes reveals that martial arts training creates measurable neuroplasticity—structural changes in the brain. In 2018, Fatih Uygur et al. released a study using Voxel-Based Morphometry (VBM) on the athletes that found increased gray matter volume in the right inferior temporal area, which is part of visual movement perception, formed through motor learning. Not just "getting better at fighting." Your brain is physically reorganizing itself to support the skills you're developing in measurable ways.

Neuroplasticity is the ability of the brain to change and adapt throughout a person's life by forming new neural pathways, strengthening existing ones, and pruning old ones. Martial arts training creates new connections of synapses in your brain. In this way the practitioner of the arts literally reprograms themselves and the longer they train, the greater the hand they have in forming their brains structure and capabilities.

The repetition required in martial arts training—drilling the same technique hundreds, then thousands of times—creates what we call muscle memory. But it's not just your muscles learning. The repetition of techniques helps enhance memory retention and cognitive function, while martial arts training demands concentration that strengthens the prefrontal cortex—the area of the brain responsible for attention and focus.

This constant reorganization of your brain's neural pathways is precisely why martial arts training transfers to every other area of your life. The discipline you build on the mat doesn't stay on the mat—it follows you home, to work, into your relationships.

Here's exactly where, *and why*, most people fail: they expect transformation to happen faster than it actually does.

Habit Creation

You've probably heard that it takes 21 days to form a habit—False. The 21-day claim originated from anecdotal evidence of plastic surgery patients who had reportedly adjusted psychologically to their new appearance within 21 days—yes, a marketing ploy, it has no basis in habit formation analysis.

The reality is more demanding but also more honest. Most

habits take about two months to feel automatic—not three weeks. Some take even longer, up to almost a year depending on what you're trying to build.

Brief 21-day challenges or kick-starts are unlikely to be sufficient to firmly ingrain new habits—individuals should anticipate a time-frame of at least two months to develop automaticity in new health habits. You become what you do, if you do it ten thousand times.

Here is why it is actually good news. It means you can stop beating yourself up for not being "transformed" after three weeks of training. It means the struggle you're experiencing is normal, expected, and part of the process.

Scientific inquiry shows that practicing the habit in the same place and at the same time each day helps reinforce it, while early repetitions have the biggest impact on making an action feel automatic. Here is why martial arts training is so effective—you show up to the same place, at the same time, and repeat the same fundamental movements until they become second nature.

How to Build Unbreakable Discipline

Discipline isn't built through willpower alone. It's built through process, through systems, through structured repetition. One step at a time.

Many think discipline is about forcing yourself to do things you hate through sheer mental toughness. That's exhausting and unsustainable. Real discipline is about designing a system so appealing that following it becomes easier than not following it. It's about creating joyful momentum that carries you forward even when motivation fails.

Let me give you the outline. It's simple in principle but demands precision in execution.

Think of achieving any major goal as a mathematical equation—but don't worry, this is the only math you need to

know: You take daily steps that hit specific benchmarks, and you do this consistently over time until you reach your objective. Steps plus benchmarks over time equals objective. That's it. That's the entire formula.

Let me break down what each piece actually means in practice.

Steps are the specific actions you take every single day. Not "train harder" or "eat better." Concrete actions: fifty pushups before breakfast. Ten minutes of drilling footwork. Two rounds of shadowboxing before bed. These are your daily essentials—the tasks that, when completed, move you measurably closer to where you want to be.

Benchmarks are the checkpoints that prove you're on track. These are small goals set and achieved along the journey. If your ultimate objective is a black belt, your benchmarks might be: learn all yellow belt forms within two months, successfully defend against a larger opponent by month four, execute twenty perfect roundhouse kicks in a row by month six. Benchmarks are the evidence that your daily steps are working. They're also psychological fuel—each one you hit proves to yourself that you're capable of the next one.

Time is your schedule, your commitment to consistency. We aren't just marking days on a calendar. It's the sacred agreement you make with yourself about when and how often you'll show up. Four times per week, Tuesday through Friday, six to seven-thirty PM, no exceptions. Time is the container that holds everything else. Without it, steps are just random actions and benchmarks are just wishes.

The objective is your North Star—the final accomplishment you're aiming for. Not a fuzzy dream, but a specific, measurable goal that you can definitively achieve or not achieve. "Get better at martial arts" isn't an objective. "Earn a black belt in Brazilian Jiu-Jitsu within three years" is an objective. "Compete in a tournament" isn't specific enough. "Win a medal at the regional championships in the under-185-pound division by next November" is an objective. The clearer your objective, the easier it is to reverse-engineer the benchmarks and steps that will get you there.

Now let me show you how to actually build this system, piece by piece.

First, you must set a grand objective that's specific enough to be real.

Not "get better at martial arts." That's too vague to be useful. You need something you can see in your mind with perfect clarity: earn a black belt in Tae Kwon Do. Compete in your first tournament and not get submitted in the first round. Master the flying arm-bar. Develop the conditioning to spar five full rounds without gassing out.

The objective has to be ambitious enough to excite you but specific enough that you'll know the moment you achieve it. There's no ambiguity. Either you have the black belt or you don't. Either you lasted five rounds or you didn't. This clarity is essential because vague goals produce vague effort.

Once you know exactly where you're going, you work backward to identify every step required to get there.

A common failing point is setting a big goal but never breaking it down into the actual work required. Let's say your objective is earning a black belt. Ask yourself: What needs to happen daily? What techniques must I master? What physical conditioning benchmarks must I hit? What tests must I pass? What knowledge must I acquire?

Daily, you might need: one hour of technical training, thirty minutes of conditioning, fifteen minutes of meditation or visualization. Weekly, you might need: two sparring sessions, one private lesson, review of video footage from training. Monthly, you might need: test preparation for the next belt level, competing in a local tournament to pressure-test your skills, meeting with your instructor to assess progress and identify weak points.

Write it all down. Every single component. If your goal is a black belt and that typically takes five years, you're looking at roughly sixty belt tests, hundreds of techniques to master, thousands of hours of training. Break it into pieces small enough that you can see exactly what you need to do tomorrow morning. This is easily transferable to any goal you set in your life. A promotion, a new car, 10 pounds of weight loss. Master the formula, and the plan writes itself.

Then—and this is critical—you make every action in your entire day serve the objective.

Your whole life becomes aligned with where you're going. Run up stairs instead of walking. Hop down them to condition your legs and improve your balance. Practice footwork while you're waiting in line at the grocery store. Visualize techniques before you sleep—your mind drilling the movements while your body rests. Stretch while watching TV. Do wall sits during phone calls.

Every moment is either moving you toward your goal or away from it. There is no neutral. When you choose to skip the morning workout, you're not just staying the same—you're actively moving backward because your competition didn't skip theirs. When you choose to eat clean instead of grabbing fast food, you're not just avoiding harm—you're building an advantage.

This might sound extreme, but here's the truth: your competitors are doing this whether you know it or not. The person who will beat you for that tournament spot is practicing footwork in line at Starbucks right now. The person who will earn their black belt while you're still stuck at brown is visualizing techniques before bed every single night. You're not competing against some abstract standard—you're competing against real people who want it as badly as you do and might be willing to work harder for it.

Next, you create a calendar with pre-planned milestones and you make it visible.

Start today. Get a physical calendar or a detailed digital one. Record weekly goals and monthly benchmarks. Make them specific and measurable: "Master the rear naked choke escape by February 15th." "Complete a five-mile run in under forty minutes by March 1st." "Successfully execute the tornado kick three times in a row by April 10th."

Update the calendar as you meet each milestone. Check them off. See the progress accumulate. This visual evidence of forward momentum is psychologically essential when motivation dips—and motivation will dip. On the morning when you don't feel like training, when you're tired and sore and questioning why you're doing this, you can look at that calendar and see twenty benchmarks you already crushed. That's proof you're the kind of person who keeps their commitments.

Consider adding personal rewards when you hit major milestones. Not to bribe yourself, but to acknowledge progress and create positive reinforcement. Hit your six-month conditioning benchmark? Buy that new gi you've been wanting. Master all the yellow belt forms two weeks early? Take yourself out for a nice meal. Small celebrations matter—they mark the journey and give you moments to appreciate how far you've come before pushing toward the next challenge.

Then you build in regular review and adjustment—because no plan survives contact with reality unchanged.

Pick a consistent time. Maybe Sunday mornings at six AM with coffee. Maybe Friday evenings after your last training session of the week. The specific time matters less than the consistency. The plan is to sit down and honestly assess: What's working? What's not? Where are the gaps in my development?

Maybe you're hitting all your technical benchmarks but your cardio is falling behind. Adjust. Add two extra conditioning sessions per week. Maybe your footwork is sharp but you're getting caught in the same submission repeatedly. Identify the problem, find a coach or training partner who can help you address it specifically, and drill the counter until it becomes automatic.

Sometimes you realize you need different training partners to push you harder. Sometimes you need a new environment—a different gym, a different class time, a different instructor with fresh perspective. Sometimes you discover that a benchmark you set was unrealistic given your current commitments, and you need to adjust the timeline without abandoning the objective.

This regular review keeps you honest. It forces you to confront the gap between where you planned to be and where you actually are. And then—applying the warrior's mindset—it demands that you problem-solve instead of making excuses.

Finally, you execute this system with one simple rule: achieve today's goals, then adjust tomorrow based on what you learned today.

Stay flexible in your tactics while remaining completely committed to your strategy. The objective doesn't change—you're still earning that black belt, you're still competing in that tournament, you're still mastering that technique. But the path to get there might shift based on what you discover along the way.

Maybe you planned to drill guard passes for an hour but you're nursing a shoulder injury. Fine. Adjust. Spend that hour drilling guard retention instead—work from bottom position where your shoulder isn't stressed. You stayed committed to training, you just modified the specific technique based on current reality.

Maybe you planned to spar five rounds but you're getting destroyed by everyone in the gym tonight. Your ego wants you to keep going, to prove something. But your strategic mind says: "I'm exhausted, my technique is sloppy, I'm not learning anything useful right now, and I'm risking injury." So you adjust. You bow out after three rounds, you go drill fundamentals for thirty minutes instead, and tomorrow you come back fresh and sharp.

This flexibility is not weakness—it's intelligence. Rigid tactics break under pressure. Adaptive tactics bend and flow and ultimately prevail. The objective remains fixed. The path evolves.

Let me show you this system in action with a real example.

Imagine your objective is to compete in your first Brazilian Jiu-Jitsu tournament six months from now and not get submitted in the first minute. That's specific. That's measurable. It is ambitious, but achievable.

You work backward. To not get submitted immediately, you need solid defensive fundamentals: escapes from mount, side control, back control. You need submission defense for the most common attacks: armbar, triangle, rear naked choke, guillotine. You need decent cardio so you don't gas out in the first round.

Your benchmarks over six months might be: Month one—master the basic trap and roll escape from mount. Month two—defend successfully against arm-bars from guard ten times in a row during drilling. Month three—escape side control against a resisting opponent of similar skill. Month four—survive five-minute rolls with upper belts without getting submitted. Month five—successfully defend all basic submissions in live sparring. Month six—compete in a smaller in-house tournament for pressure-test experience before the real event.

Your daily steps: show up to class four times per week. Drill escapes every single session for at least fifteen minutes. Roll with at least two different people each class. Run twice a week to build cardio. Watch instructional videos of the specific techniques you're working on. Visualize the tournament before bed—see yourself calm, technical, defensive, surviving.

You create a calendar. You mark every benchmark. And then you start executing.

Three months in, during your regular Sunday review, you realize you're hitting all your technical benchmarks but you're panicking when people get heavy top pressure. Your technique disappears under the weight. So you adjust. You seek out the biggest, heaviest training partners specifically and ask them to work from top position. You drill staying calm under pressure. You're not changing the objective—you're adapting your tactics to address a specific weakness you discovered.

Six months later, you step onto the mat for your first tournament. You don't win. But you don't get submitted in thirty seconds either. You survive the first round using the escapes you drilled a thousand times. You lose on points, but you competed. You proved to yourself that your system works. And now you're ready to set the next objective: win your next match. And you already know how to build the system to get there.

That's how discipline is built—not through superhuman willpower, but through systematic execution of a well-designed plan.

Steps plus benchmarks over time equals objective. Do the daily work. Hit the checkpoints. Stay consistent over time. Adjust as needed. Keep your eyes on the finish line.

The formula is simple, although not easy or comfortable. The execution demands your everything. But when you apply this system with warrior discipline, success becomes inevitable.

And that's the difference between someone who dreams about a black belt and someone who earns one.

Training Until Learning Occurs

When you walk, eat, or sleep, yourself performs these actions automatically. It knows exactly what to do and requires no input from the mind. The result of martial arts training is techniques executed without thought, responses that happen faster than conscious decision-making allows, body over mind.

Think about walking up stairs. If you overthink the approach, the gait, the step speed, it becomes awkward. Your conscious mind interferes with what your body already knows. It should be an easy automatic action, but overthinking is the enemy of action. This act should be one of sub conscious memorization. It is a program that you run on without thought. Repetition training locks in that program.

Brawler or Fighter

One element of discipline that separates trained fighters from brawlers is the ability to accurately break down a combat interaction play by play.

After sparring, a trained martial artist can tell you: what happened, what went right, what went wrong, and what needs work. Being able to verbalize what needs improvement in yourself is difficult, but with practice and presence—being hyper-aware during contact with an adversary—you learn to identify areas for improvement and your opponent's weaknesses.

If you can learn to do this fast enough, you can do it while you're in combat.

The distinction between a trained fighter and a brawler isn't in at its core genetic talent or toughness — it's two totally different approaches. The brawler operates on assumption. They believe that what they naturally possess will be sufficient when the moment arrives. Sometimes it is. More often it isn't. And because they have no system, they have no way to diagnose why they lost or what to correct before the next encounter.

The fighter operates differently. They understand that performance is the accumulated product of preparation, and that preparation is measured not in single heroic efforts but in consistency over time. Three variables compound directly into outcome: showing up to every scheduled session without exception, bringing full effort to each one, and extracting a lesson from every experience — wins, losses, and the unremarkable sessions in between. Each is a concrete input that either improves your baseline or allows it to erode.

Think of it in mechanical terms. Your nervous system, your conditioning, your technique — these are programs running on biological hardware. Like any program, they execute according to what was written into them. Inconsistent training writes incomplete code. Full-effort training without reflection writes fast but flawed code. The fighter who trains consistently, works at maximum capacity, and actively processes what they're learning is writing clean, tested, reliable code — the kind that runs under pressure without crashing.

The brawler has no program. They have instincts, some physical attributes, and a willingness to engage. Against an untrained opponent, that may be sufficient. Against someone who has spent years debugging their own performance, it rarely is.

Discipline, in this context, isn't a character trait you either have or don't. It's the operational habit of protecting your training variables from the interference of convenience, fatigue, and circumstance. The fighter who treats their schedule as negotiable has already introduced error into the system — and errors accumulate.

When related to fighting or war, the ultimate goal is predictable outcomes. If you must fight, you want to win—every time, with minimal self-damage while inflicting exactly the right amount of damage necessary to win. This happens when there is strict discipline in training and execution of tactics and techniques. Repeat what you want to happen in practice over and over until all the bugs are worked out and you are always nailing it. Fighters know this and train and train some more. Brawlers rely on luck, and hope what they have naturally will be enough for the win. The battlefield is no place to run on luck and gamble with losing.

The fighter knows that science supports his disciplined methods, testing new techniques in a training environment and continually drilling what works. The neuroplasticity of your brain and its encoded muscle memory dictate that the more you do something, the more resources develop to support the activity. Conversely, the less you do something, the less capable your consciousness and body become at performing the task.

This means you're either building capacity or losing it. There's no maintenance mode. You're either moving forward or sliding backward.

Dedication equals discipline. Perseverance equals discipline. Focus equals discipline.

Be responsible to yourself for all that is in your realm of control. Take charge of your training goals and schedule the game plan. Make daily lists and cross off accomplishments with pride. Attack your goals with passion and purpose. Dream big and shoot for the stars—you will make it further than you can possibly imagine. Make your first goal 90 days of daily training. Attend and check it off the list each day.

But understand what this requires: Grit. Not being pampered, entitled, self-absorbed, or emotionally delicate. Grit means showing up when it's hard. Grit means continuing when others quit. Grit means refusing to make excuses. Grit is what a winning warrior is made of.

Those who lift themselves up by their own efforts, who better themselves and in turn make the world around them better—these people earn respect. Those who take personal responsibility for their development, who don't wait for perfect conditions or external motivation—these are the people who transform.

Waiting for the right time is how you waste your life. The time is now.

You Will be Tested

The fight that's coming for you—it might be a physical altercation. It might be a career challenge, a relationship struggle, a health crisis, a moment where you're tested in ways you can't predict.

What matters is that when it arrives, you're ready. Not because you got lucky. Not because the work was easy. But because you prepared through disciplined training, day after day, when nobody was watching and when it didn't feel glamorous.

Martial arts training is the proving ground for this personal discipline. It's where you learn that a lazy mind gives up long before the body fails. It's where you discover that consistency compounds into capability. It's where you build the kind of discipline that earns your own respect. Once you have the formula, you can apply it everywhere to any challenge and see positive results quickly.

In the next chapter, we'll discuss how to choose the martial art that serves your goals, fits your life, and provides the structure for this transformative discipline to take root.

But first, you need to make a decision: Will you commit to the disciplined path? Will you show up, not when it's convenient, but because it's necessary? Will you do the work that transforms a white belt into a black belt, not through shortcuts, but through the daily practice that rewires your brain and rebuilds your character? Do you want to gamble like a brawler, or win like a warrior?

The fight is coming. The only question is whether you'll be ready.

CHAPTER 2 – EMBRACE A STYLE

"If you want to be a lion, train with lions."—Carlson Gracie, 1979

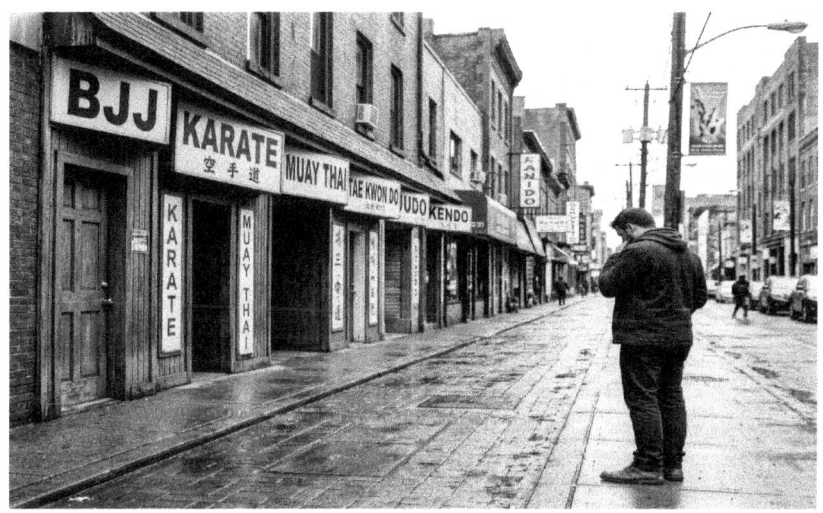

M ost people who decide to train in martial arts quit within six months. Not because the training is too hard—though it is hard—but because they chose the wrong art, the wrong school, or the wrong instructor at the wrong time in their lives. Being inspired to train diligently relies on the fusion of the right elements: a good school, the right master, and a little luck with timing.

Here's the truth: martial arts are varied in scope and style, but they will all bring you to a place of health, general wellness, clarity, and physical capability. Every legitimate martial art—whether striking or grappling, traditional or modern, weapons-based or empty-hand—offers a path to transformation. The question isn't which art is "best." The question is which art is best for you.

Choosing a martial art isn't like picking a gym membership. You're not just selecting a workout routine. You're choosing a philosophy, a community, and a path of development that will reshape how you move through the world. The difference between the right choice and the wrong one is the difference between transformation and frustration, between a lifelong practice and another abandoned New Year's resolution.

A 'martial artist' is a person having an affinity for, and skilled in warlike techniques. They can display and perform this knowledge with practiced precision. An artist is not just "doing techniques." They express them. Each movement is an interpretation of codified wisdom passed down through generations of masters, filtered through culture and combat experience, all captured within the confines and capabilities of the human body. A practitioner takes traditional movements and personalizes the corporeal defense and attack exercises, deciphering and enacting them in their own unique expressive way—where the martial move becomes art.

To become a martial artist in your own right, you will first need to find your art.

This chapter will guide you through that choice. We'll examine the major categories of martial arts—what they emphasize, what they demand, and what they develop. We'll discuss how to evaluate schools and instructors, how to identify red flags and green lights, and how to match your temperament, goals, and life circumstances to the right training environment. We'll cover the difference between traditional and modern approaches, the value of lineage versus innovation, and why the instructor matters more than the style.

By the end, you'll have the details for making an informed decision—one that leads not to six months of attendance followed by quiet disappearance, but to years of growth, challenge, and the transformation that comes from committing to something bigger than comfort.

It takes a village to raise a child, and a skilled master to hone a warrior. Let's find yours.

Know Yourself First

Let's establish your personal attributes as they apply to which art is ideal. Before you walk into any dojo or gym, before you sign up for a single class, we need to have an honest conversation. I'm going to ask you four questions. Your answers will determine whether you thrive in martial arts training or quit after six weeks of frustration.

These aren't casual questions. They require real introspection, the kind most people avoid because it forces them to confront uncomfortable truths about themselves. But choosing the wrong martial art because you didn't do this self-assessment first is like buying expensive running shoes when what you actually need is a bicycle. The equipment might be excellent, but it's solving the wrong problem.

So let's get honest. Grab a pen if you need to. Think carefully. And don't give me the answer you think sounds impressive—give me the truth.

Question One: What is your primary goal?

Be brutally specific here. "Get better at fighting" is completely different from "learn self-defense." "Get in shape" is different from "compete in tournaments." Your goal determines everything else—the art you choose, the school you attend, even how you measure progress. Know the goal, know the journey.

Let me break down the most common goals so you can identify yours. If your primary driver is self-defense, you need practical, efficient techniques that work under stress against untrained attackers. Hours matter more than years here. You're not preparing for a tournament with rules and weight classes—you're preparing for the parking lot, the home invasion, the unexpected violence that gives you no warning. This means you need **reality-based training, scenario work, and techniques** that function when you're scared, tired, or caught off guard.

Maybe your real goal is physical fitness. You want a demanding workout that builds strength, endurance, and confidence. The martial aspect is honestly secondary to the physical transformation. That's completely legitimate, but it changes what you're looking for. You need high-intensity training with lots of drilling, conditioning, and physical challenges. The traditional ceremony and philosophy? Less important. You want to leave every class drenched in sweat and feeling accomplished.

Or perhaps you're drawn to traditional culture—the ceremony, history, and philosophy embedded in classical arts. The spiritual dimension matters as much as the physical. You're fascinated by the lineage, the formal etiquette, the meditation practices. You want to bow in and out of class, learn the Japanese or Chinese terminology, understand the deeper meaning behind the movements. This is about personal development through ancient wisdom, not just learning how to punch.

Then there's competition. You want to test yourself against others, win medals, prove your skill in the arena. You need an art with an active competitive scene and instructors who understand the fighter's path—the training regimen, the mental preparation, the tactical analysis of opponents. You're not interested in self-defense scenarios or spiritual growth. You want the adrenaline rush of the match, the clarity of win or lose, the measurable progress of climbing the ranks.

And finally, there's mental health and well-being. Maybe you're dealing with stress, anxiety, anger issues, or depression. A systematic review of martial arts training found medium-to-large positive effects on anxiety and depression, with meaningful improvements in overall well-being. Comparing martial arts practitioners to athletes in other sports, researchers found that karate and jujitsu students showed lower levels of verbal hostility and aggressive behavior compared to students in rugby and badminton clubs. If mental health is driving your search, you need an art that emphasizes meditation, controlled aggression, and the psychological benefits of disciplined training.

Most people want some combination of these goals. That's normal. But one drives the others. One is the core motivation that will get you to class when you don't feel like going. Identify it clearly. Write it down. This becomes your North Star when choosing an art.

Once you know your goal, the second question becomes: Where are you in life?

Your age, physical condition, and life circumstances matter enormously. A sixteen-year-old has completely different needs than a thirty-five-year-old father of three. Both can train effectively, but they need different approaches.

Start with your physical attributes. Most people are more coordinated with their hands than their feet—that's just basic human biomechanics. Some of you are naturally flexible, others are stiff but strong. Longer limbs favor striking range and create distance advantages. Shorter, stockier builds often excel in grappling where leverage and center of gravity matter more than reach. Understanding your physical starting point helps you choose an art that works with your body, not against it.

Then consider the threats you're most likely to face at your current life stage. Young children need coordination and socialization more than practical self-defense. Teenagers face schoolyard confrontations, chokes against lockers, and increasingly, awareness of weapons in school environments. College-aged adults encounter bar fights, alcohol-fueled aggression, and social violence. Adults need practical self-defense that works when you're out of shape, rusty, carrying groceries, or holding a child's hand. The techniques that work for a fit twenty-year-old don't necessarily work for a forty-year-old with a bad knee and thirty extra pounds.

Finally, be honest about time and recovery. A seventeen-year-old can train hard six days a week, get beat up in sparring, and bounce back the next morning ready for more. A forty-year-old with a career and family needs an art that builds the body rather than breaks it. You can't afford to be injured for weeks because you pushed too hard. You need training that's sustainable over decades, not just months.

Now comes the hardest question—Question Three: What are your weaknesses?

I need you to be ruthless here because your weaknesses will determine whether you succeed or quit. Ask yourself these hard questions and demand honest answers:

Are you afraid of being hit in the face? Some people freeze at the first punch. Others don't. If you're in the first category, you can choose a striking art that forces you to confront this fear head-on until it dissolves, or you can choose a grappling art where face punches are rare. Both approaches work. But you need to know which you're choosing.

Are you uncomfortable with close physical contact? Grappling arts require you to be chest-to-chest, tangled up, sweating on each other. If that makes your skin crawl, acknowledge it. You can work through it, or you can choose a striking art with more distance. But denying the discomfort won't make it disappear.

Are you lacking upper body strength? Many arts rely heavily on it. If you're weak there, you either need to build that strength first or choose an art that emphasizes technique over power—leverage-based arts where a smaller person can control a larger opponent through positioning rather than muscle.

Are you inflexible? High kicks and deep stances might frustrate you initially. Again, you can work on flexibility over time, or you can choose an art where it matters less. Both paths are valid.

Here's where it gets psychologically complex: Are you quick to anger or overly aggressive? Some people are. They need an art that teaches control and channels that aggression productively. Conversely, are you passive and conflict-avoidant? You might need an art that builds assertiveness and comfort with confrontation.

The key insight here is this: you can choose an art that addresses your weaknesses head-on, forcing you to develop in areas where you're deficient. Or you can choose an art that lets you develop around your weaknesses, playing to your strengths. Both approaches work. But you need to consciously know which path you're taking. The worst outcome is choosing an art randomly and then quitting because it exposes a weakness you weren't prepared to face.

That brings us to the final question—Question

Four: What will you actually stick with?

This is the most important question of all, and it's the one most people ignore. Here's the brutal truth: the "best" martial art is completely worthless if you hate training and quit after three months. The art you'll train in four times a week for years is infinitely more valuable than the objectively "perfect" art you'll train in twice a month before giving up.

Kendo is completely different from Judo. They appeal to different people for different reasons. Some people love the meditative focus of kata and forms. Others find them boring and crave the chaos of live sparring. Some thrive in the individual challenge of one-on-one combat. Others need the camaraderie of group training and team energy.

Think about what actually motivates you. Do you need social connection to stay consistent, or do you prefer training alone? Do you get bored with repetition, or does ritual comfort you? Do you need immediate feedback and visible progress, or can you trust the long-term process? Are you self-motivated, or do you need external accountability?

Your personal attributes—your answers to these four questions—will narrow which arts fit into your realm of possibility. Don't fight your nature. Work with it. Examine specifically the arts that match your natural inclinations as described by your answers.

Now let me give you an example of how this works in practice.

Imagine a thirty-two-year-old woman—let's call her Sarah. She's got two young kids, works full-time, and hasn't been in a fight since elementary school. When Sarah answers these four questions honestly, here's what emerges:

Her primary goal is self-defense after a close call in a parking lot left her feeling vulnerable. She's in decent shape but not athletic. She's inflexible and uncomfortable with the idea of getting punched in the face, but she's determined. She has maybe three hours a week to train, and she needs something that won't leave her too injured to take care of her kids.

Based on these answers, Sarah doesn't need Muay Thai with heavy sparring six days a week. She'd quit after the first bloody nose. She doesn't need traditional Tai Chi focused on forms and philosophy. She'd get frustrated at the slow pace when what she really wants is practical skills now. What Sarah needs is a reality-based self-defense program or a Brazilian Jiu-Jitsu fundamentals class—something practical, scalable to her schedule, focused on technique over athleticism, and building real capability without requiring her to get punched repeatedly.

Do you see how the four questions led to a clear answer? That's what I want for you. Not a random choice based on what school is closest or what your friend happens to do. A deliberate choice based on honest self-assessment.

Different Styles for Different Stages

Over the years and depending where I was located, I've trained in Kung-fu, Shotokan, Tae Kwon Do, MMA, Brazilian Jiu-Jitsu, and boxing. I also tested and trialed many other forms as the opportunities presented themselves. Each taught me something different. Each had its place in my development. Here's what you need to know about the major mainstream martial arts, not from theory, but from the mat.

A young child (8–12) benefits from arts that develop coordination and respect for tradition—Tae Kwon Do, or Karate, emphasize kicking techniques that train the mind's control over the extremities and instills discipline through belt systems and formal etiquette. These types of styles are best for beginners and younger people. It's your entry into the fighting ring and organized competition.

What it teaches: How to take a blow and give one back. How to perform in front of audiences during tournaments. The mental game of competition without the intimidation factor of getting punched in the face repeatedly.

The limitation is obvious—striking is very leg-based and tends toward the flashy. But here's what most critics miss: using your legs and transferring weight through the hips builds the most power. Most people are not as coordinated with their feet as with their hands. Train your feet intensively and you gain an advantage over practitioners of other arts who neglect leg techniques. When everyone else is hand-fighting, you have weapons they've never properly developed.

Teenagers (13-18) have the energy and resilience for intense grappling, and kickboxing. Wrestling builds toughness, teaches you to impose your will on a resisting opponent, and develops a base that serves any future martial arts training.

Wrestling and kickboxing offers young teens a dynamic combination of physical and psychological benefits during a crucial developmental stage. The sport builds cardiovascular endurance, coordination, and functional strength while teaching proper body mechanics that reduce injury risk in other activities. Beyond the physical gains, kickboxing instills discipline and focus—teens learn to follow instruction, practice techniques with precision, and work toward progressive skill milestones. The structured environment provides a healthy outlet for adolescent energy and stress while building genuine self-confidence rooted in acquired competence rather than empty praise.

Whether wrestling or kickboxing, training alongside peers creates a supportive community where teens develop respect, sportsmanship, and communication skills. Perhaps most valuable during these formative years, these physical outlets teaches teens that improvement comes through consistent effort and that setbacks are simply part of the learning process. This growth mindset, combined with basic self-defense awareness, equips young people with both the physical capability and mental foundation to navigate challenges with confidence and resilience.

But this age group requires careful attention. Male martial artists are particularly prone to injury during adolescence, with injury rates peaking at age 14. The common hyper extended knee or elbow ligaments can linger for many years, for example. This isn't an argument against training—it's an argument for proper supervision and progressive intensity.

Young adults (18-25) can handle the demands of mixed martial arts (MMA) or combat sports like Muay Thai or Brazilian Jiu-Jitsu (BJJ). These arts teach you what actually works under pressure. One class of Muay Thai will teach you more about real fighting than a year in many traditional arts—not because traditional arts are worthless, but because combat sports cut through the BS.

MMA mixes all skill sets, and that's where you discover what actually works when the rules open up. MMA has by far the greatest range and most realistic style. It is directly transferable to street fighting. Pick this if you have the desire for intense physical challenge. Muay Thai is the base for the majority of striking techniques used in MMA and it is a style that many champion fighters claim as their origin art. Expect rock hard shins with devastating knees and elbows to be your tools of choice in this style.

In striking, the hardest, most direct hit ends a fight. In BJJ, the smarter fighter has the advantage. You learn patience. You learn that dominating position matters more than explosive action. You learn that technique can overcome significant size and strength disadvantages—to a point.

In BJJ, anaerobic strength and endurance matter as much as aerobic capacity. Balance doesn't always favor the stronger competitor. The game can be won by outmaneuvering rather than overpowering. You can stall advances, suffocate your opponent's options, and wither their will to fight on.

During a match, understanding and evaluating your opponent's strengths and weaknesses becomes the key to winning. You must not let them fight their fight. Keep them in their weakest place. A pure striker who can't grapple? Take them down. Fighting a BJJ specialist and have no takedown defense? Distance + damage + sprawl–when–forced = victory. Rushing in? Angle off and counter — do not move backwards in straight lines, watch for the opportunity to push the head down and apply a guillotine.

Adults in their prime (25–45) often benefit from returning to traditional arts like Kung Fu and Karate. These provide demanding training within a philosophical underpinning that becomes more meaningful with life experience. They keep you in peak condition while teaching principles that extend beyond the mat.

Later in life (45+), less contact arts like <u>Tai Chi</u>, or <u>Aikido</u> offer continued development without the wear and tear of hard sparring. They emphasize efficiency, biomechanics, and the mental aspects of martial arts. And here's something that surprises most people: injury data from properly supervised martial arts programs shows that older adults actually sustain fewer training injuries than younger practitioners. Intense martial arts training for older adults presented significant functional fitness improvements—strength gains of 9–34%, mobility improvements of 10–14%, and balance improvements of over 20%. The fear that you're "too old" for martial arts is largely unfounded.

These are possible paths—not prescriptions. You might start Brazilian Jiu–Jitsu at 40 and thrive. The point is that your training can evolve as you do.

YiQuan; the Visualization Style

There are an incredible array of arts globally and there is truly an art for everybody no matter how or what specifics you want to develop. As we examine martial arts throughout this book, visualization and meditation will continue to be emphasized as powerful, irreplaceable tools you must employ.

One art, Yiquan (Mind Boxing), uses almost solely a meditative state to train. Developed 100 years ago in Beijing, YiQuan uses visualization as its core focus to generate explosive power from minimal movement.

Through standing meditation (zhan zhuang) and subtle tensing exercises, practitioners mentally simulate combat scenarios while remaining nearly motionless. By intensely focusing on internal sensations—imagining pressure like hot water flowing through the body—they gradually gain conscious control over muscle groups normally beyond voluntary command, including deep stabilizers and even organ tissue.

This hyper-awareness allows practitioners to recruit their *entire* muscular system simultaneously during strikes or when absorbing blows. Where untrained fighters use only surface muscles, Yiquan practitioners engage everything from skin to sinew to core, creating disproportionate power from compact movements.

The visualization acts as a neural trigger: the mind rehearses scenarios so thoroughly that the body's conditioned response becomes automatic in actual combat. Like resilience training where gradually increasing strikes build absorption capacity, mental rehearsal builds whole-body coordination and hardening on demand. (Pavlovian conditioning)

The result: devastating power generated not through large movements, but through total-body integration activated in an instant.

Yiquan is just an example of the multitude of martial arts

available to you. Perhaps you will be inspired to seek out an aged master of an obscure art to train with in the mountains of Tibet. Variety is the spice of life, and I recommend to explore and seek your type of spicy.

Skip the Wait: Which Art Is Best?

Here's the truth that will disappoint people looking for simple answers: the why is more important than the which.

Each new student enters martial training for different reasons. Some want to defend themselves. Some want to compete and win. Some want discipline and structure. Some want to lose weight and gain confidence. Some are searching for something they can't even name yet.

I want each person to find success in their initial goal, plus many more benefits they'll be surprised to discover as bonuses. That's what martial arts training delivers when you choose the right art for your purpose.

Fighting and winning fights has too many variables to declare one art supreme. Cultural context matters—what works in a ring with rules doesn't always work in a back alley without them. Climate affects technique—try doing spinning kicks on ice. Body shape and nutrition determine what you can execute effectively. The environment alters options: a cage, a ring, a street, a confined space, each demands different approaches. Weapons availability varies by geographic location and setting—an art that ignores weapons entirely leaves you unprepared for most real-world violence.

So when someone asks me, "Which martial art is best?" I ask them: Best for what? Best for whom? Best when and where?

A 50-year-old businessman who wants fitness and stress relief doesn't need the same art as a 20-year-old who wants to compete in the cage. A woman concerned about sexual assault needs different training than a bouncer dealing with drunk men. A high school kid being bullied has different requirements than a law enforcement officer.

The "best" martial art is the one that serves your goals, fits your body and life circumstances, and—critically—that you'll actually train in consistently for years.

Everything else is ego and marketing.

Pick it and Stick it

There's a time and place for cross-training, and a time to specialize.

Early in your development, pick one art and commit. Model the instructors precisely. Get competent, then proficient, then skilled. Once you have a solid base—and I mean years of training, not months—then consider adding another dimension. Bouncing from art to art or training in multiple styles simultaneously is counter productive.

Striking and grappling are essentially opposite disciplines and require completely different training approaches. Your body adapts differently. Your mindset shifts. A striker learns to maintain distance and deliver damage from range. A grappler learns to close distance and control through contact.

The danger of cross-training too early is becoming mediocre at everything instead of excellent at something. The benefit of cross-training once you have a base is discovering the gaps in your game and becoming more complete.

MMA fighters understand this. The best ones aren't equally good at everything—they're elite at one or two things and competent enough in the rest to avoid being exploited. A majority of their early years tended to be rooted to one style before they widened their scope of training.

There's a logical progression to martial arts training that follows human development. A proper sequential curriculum. There should be a logic to the training—a building-block process where each class compounds your understanding. One exercise leads to another for a reason. When you assemble all the pieces, there's a cohesive, operable, interconnected set of skills available on tap.

Popular Club in your Area

For your first foray into martial arts, I recommend joining a large school nearby. Not the one that sounds coolest online. Not the one Joe Rogan talks about. The one that's actually thriving where you live.

Why? A large teaching cadre and many training partners ensures you will integrate smoother. With a large variety of personalities it is easier to find friends who you click with. Martial arts training creates bonds that other activities don't. You're literally trusting people not to hurt you too badly, while you practice hurting each other. You're pushing through exhaustion together. You're showing up when it's hard. Having reliable partners to embark this journey with, will help to cement your regular attendance.

A popular local school solves several problems simultaneously. It gives you a reliable pool of training partners for drilling outside of class. It provides people who understand the specific demands of what you're doing — the schedule, the soreness, the plateaus — without requiring explanation. And it creates the social infrastructure that keeps you showing up when the novelty has worn off, which research consistently identifies as the primary reason people abandon training programs: not difficulty, but the absence of social accountability.

Before you commit to any school, watch a class. Not a promotional tour — an actual class. You're looking at four things that reveal the real culture of a school more accurately than any website or sales conversation. How students treat each other during drilling — whether there's patience or contempt toward people learning slower. The intensity and focus during rounds, not just during the instructor's demonstration. Whether advanced students engage with beginners or cluster exclusively among themselves. And the general atmosphere — whether the room feels competitive in a productive way or in a way that makes people protective of their techniques.

That last observation matters more than most people realize. Some schools quietly discourage sharing because knowledge is treated as competitive advantage within the gym. Others operate on the understanding that everyone improves faster when everyone improves. The latter environment produces better practitioners, and you can identify it by watching how freely upper-level students coach during sparring rounds.

Your training partners will shape your development as directly as your instructor. The instructor sets the curriculum. Your partners are the laboratory where that curriculum gets tested, and the quality of that testing determines how fast you progress. A resisting opponent who genuinely challenges you forces adaptation. A passive partner who lets you succeed teaches you nothing that will hold up under real pressure. Studies on skill acquisition in contact sports consistently show that the quality of practice opposition is a stronger predictor of improvement than total training hours — meaning five hundred hours against mediocre partners produces a less capable practitioner than three hundred hours against committed ones.

Find people who arrived around the same time you did and invest in those relationships deliberately. You'll track each other's progress over years. You'll understand each other's gaps. You'll be honest with each other in ways that a more senior student might soften. That peer-level feedback, accumulated over time, is irreplaceable — and it's only available in a school with enough people training seriously that you have real options for who you work with.

More Thoughts about Teachers

Pick a teacher who is moral and honorable, that you can respect and emulate. Skills can be taught by anyone competent.

Character can only be modeled by someone who has it.

Your instructor matters more than the style. A great instructor in a "lesser" art will develop you far more than a mediocre instructor in a "superior" art.

Quality instruction pushes you to your limits and beyond. You should leave every class knowing you exerted major effort. Pain equals gain. But there's a difference between hard training and reckless training. A good instructor knows where that line is.

The best scenario is an instructor with whom you make a personal connection. Sometimes instruction is gentle, sometimes it's tough love—reminding you that your mind gives up long before your body fails. What matters is whether you can learn from this person. Can you admire them? Do they communicate in a way that reaches you?

You're not just learning techniques—you're absorbing an approach to challenge, to discipline, to dealing with ego and fear. Your instructor's character will influence yours whether you realize it or not. If they're dishonorable, you'll either absorb that or spend energy resisting it. Neither serves your development.

Look for someone whose life you'd want to emulate, not just someone who can fight well.

WARNING: You Need to Hear

I remember opening my first martial arts book, desperate to learn how to face a street fight. I tried practicing using the pictures to do the different movements. I was young. I was lost. I needed real classes with a real master. So I joined the first club I found. I made the mistake of falling into a group with an instructor who encouraged aggression and street fights. I loved it and this was my chance to prove myself, to myself. Suffice to say I got into a bad mindset, was constantly in fights, got kicked out of school, then kicked out of my house and wound up homeless, living on the streets for a few years. It took some time for me to reflect on why this happened. It was my fault 100% to be sure. But better influences might have lessened the time wasted and the damage done.

Teachers are human. They have flaws. They make mistakes. Do not idolize them.

Like me, I've seen other students blindly follow teachers into destructive patterns—bad techniques, toxic mindsets, even dangerous behavior—because they refused to see their teacher as anything less than perfect. Be choosy who you let into your life and into your mind.

School Considerations

Location isn't everything—but it is really important because it determines whether you'll be able show up four times a week while managing a busy life.

The world's best instructor teaching the perfect art for your goals is worthless if they're an hour away and you quit after two months because the commute is unsustainable.

Close enough that weather, traffic, and tired evenings can't become excuses. Close enough that you can train consistently for years, not months.

These three considerations—local popularity, instructor character, and proximity—will do more for your martial arts development than any analysis of which style is technically superior.

Once you've identified schools that meet these three criteria, it's time to evaluate them more carefully.

The McDojo Problem

The term "McDojo" exists for a reason: commercial martial arts schools that prioritize profit over authentic training have become disturbingly common. These chain operations, often bearing the name of a well-known practitioner who's expanded into multiple locations, deliver a standardized product designed for mass appeal rather than genuine martial development. While you'll certainly receive instruction, it's typically low-quality, generic training that ignores your individual needs and goals.

The real damage McDojos inflict goes beyond wasting your time and money—they actively kill interest in martial arts as a whole. Students receive belts on schedule, learn flashy choreography instead of practical fighting skills, and leave classes feeling good about themselves without ever being truly challenged. These schools prioritize customer retention over student growth, creating an environment where everyone progresses regardless of actual competence.

Warning signs include belt tests every few months with guaranteed advancement, young children wearing black belts, excessive emphasis on breaking boards rather than sparring, multi-year contracts that lock you in financially, and instructors with no verifiable competitive record or lineage. Perhaps most telling: you should leave training sessions exhausted and challenged, not comfortable and unchallenged.

McDojos reduce martial arts from a transformative life practice into a watered-down consumer experience. If a school feels more like a corporate franchise than a training hall, trust your instincts and look elsewhere.

Practical Considerations

Don't ignore the unglamorous factors:

Location: If the school is 65 minutes away, you won't train four times a week. You just won't. Find the best school you can access easily and consistently.

Schedule: Do class times fit your life? Can you realistically attend four times per week?

Cost: Quality instruction isn't free, but it shouldn't bankrupt you. Understand the full cost—monthly fees, testing fees, equipment, tournaments.

Trial period: Any legitimate school will let you observe and try a class or two before committing. If they won't, that's a red flag.

Attendance

Here's an uncomfortable truth: if you're not training at least four times a week, you're not serious. You're a hobbyist, and that's fine—but don't expect transformation from hobby-level commitment.

Four times a week, three minimum. Anything less and you won't develop muscle memory, won't build conditioning, won't internalize the lessons. The techniques won't become instinctual. You'll be starting over every session instead of building forward.

This commitment pays dividends beyond the physical. Investigations show martial arts training builds self-regulation skills that compound over time. The longer you train, the stronger your self-control and willpower become. All of life's little demons can be beaten with this will power; Sugar, sweets and junk food, partying, cigarettes, drugs and alcohol, laziness and procrastination. The martial arts is demanding enough that any of these have a marked performance detriment, you will pay if you indulge, even a little. The Arts keep you on the straight and narrow. They also give you purpose and a reason to be strict about cheating on your diet, or having one too many on the weekend, or even going to bed late. The martial arts regimen will keep a person in check 24/7 like an invisible parent over your shoulder. No fun, I know, but you will be thankful later.

Watch your ego — It will get you in trouble

There's a phenomenon in every martial art: the intermediate student who's learned enough to be dangerous but not enough to understand their limitations. In Brazilian Jiu-Jitsu, it's called "blue belt blues." In other arts, it's "green belt syndrome." You've progressed past beginner, you can handle white belts easily, and suddenly you think you're ready to test yourself against everyone.

Injuries happen when you overtrain, overreach, and pick fights you're not ready for. A good instructor will check this tendency. A good training partner will humble you when necessary. But ultimately, you need to check yourself.

Tournaments and competitions are invaluable, even if competition isn't your primary goal. One tournament is worth a hundred classes in terms of what you learn about yourself. They also keep you realistic about your progress. It is the place to hone your craft and a place you can explore what works.

There's no losing in competition. Either you win or you learn, and both are valuable. Competition reveals gaps in your technique, holes in your conditioning, and weaknesses in your mental game that no amount of regular training exposes.

More importantly, competition builds mental resilience. Martial arts practitioners consistently report that competing develops psychological strength that extends far beyond the arena. One MMA fighter explained it plainly: when your mind begs you to quit during grueling training, overriding that impulse forges toughness. Every time you push through physical discomfort on the mat, you're conditioning your mind to persist when life presents its inevitable challenges. Given how difficult life can be, we need all the resilience we can develop.

You don't have to make competition the center of your training. But if your art has a competitive component, test yourself occasionally. The lessons are irreplaceable.

Choosing the right art means choosing the right teacher at the right time in your life for the right reasons. It means finding a school close enough that you can train consistently. It means committing fully, managing your ego, and staying open to learning.

The style you choose will shape you, but remember: you're not just receiving the art—you're interpreting it, expressing it, making it yours.

Once you've mastered a martial art, you'll have a guide and mental edge in everything else you do. You'll understand the gravity of setting a goal and sticking with it. You'll know that anything can be achieved once your mind is made up and your will is strong. You'll have learned how to overcome struggles and obstacles. You'll have gained tools for building a better you.

But first, you have to embrace a style.

CHAPTER 3 – MANIFEST YOUR WARRIOR

"The warrior, for us, is one who sacrifices himself for the good of others. His task is to fight for the elderly, the defenseless, those who cannot provide for themselves, and above all, the children, who are the future of humanity." —Sitting Bull, Hunkpapa Sioux Leader. 1882

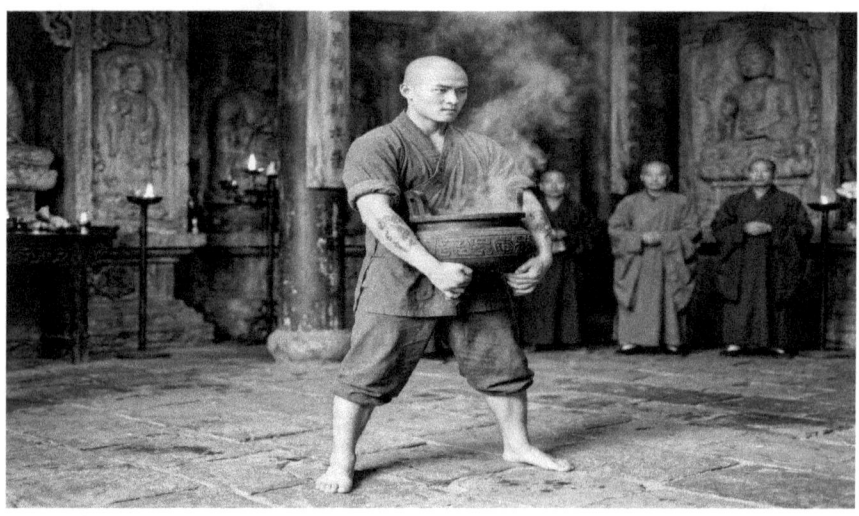

That's what separates warriors from everyone else. Not prowess alone, though that matters. Not strength of character alone, though that's essential. The warrior mindset surpasses both physicality and strong convictions.

When you have begun the journey into the martial arts you

soon realize it is the road to the warrior class of society. Train long enough and stay focused and eventually it will take you there. Transitioning from a brawler, to a fighter, to a warrior. But what is a warrior and how can one manifest it?

A warrior is someone who has forged themselves through a journey of self-development and transformed into a person of resilience, discipline, and purposeful action. A warrior proves their capabilities to themselves first, before anyone else needs to see it.

Psychological resilience represents the ability that helps people withstand emotional, cognitive, or physical difficulties. Resilience is not just the ability to bounce back from failure or challenges, but also the ability to become stronger mentally and physically and obtain superior results in the task performed.

True warriors earn universal respect through perseverance in adversity, continually improving and advancing while others give up and quit. Warriors are judged by the way they handle themselves and others while under pressure. They possess the ability to remain calm when chaos erupts, to stay mentally tough and resilient when things go wrong.

The seasoned warrior has faced both external and internal struggles. They know intuitively when to act and when to be silent. They live with courage, authenticity, and an unwavering commitment to values. They are prepared to stand up and defend what is right when necessary.

Ninja on the Mountain

There's a story that was told to me while training for competition under Master Young Lee. It's about two champions preparing for a big fight that everyone was excited to see.

The first fighter went to the biggest baddest city gym and challenged all comers. For weeks, he sparred every day and beat every challenger easily. He had no equal in the gym. He trained in the crowd, against everyone else, measuring himself by his ability to dominate those around him.

The second fighter went to the top of a mountain. He found a stream and plunged his fist into the water to catch fish. Eventually, he could catch every fish he saw. He punched and kicked trees. Internally, he challenged himself: I know I can hit harder. Could I do that faster? I know I am better than that. Throughout his training alone on the mountain, over and over he asked himself: Was that as good as I can be? Was it the best style, form, speed, and effectiveness? The voice in his head kept saying, "I know I can do better."

He trained alone, against himself.

Who won the fight?

The warrior who trained against himself. The one who refused to measure his progress by the skill level of those around him. The one who saw clearly his own weaknesses and pushed past them, sensing he could always train harder, be faster, hit with more precision.

The first fighter had become the best in his gym. He trained to the peak of others.

The second fighter had become the best version of himself. He trained to the peak of his true capability.

The warrior's path demands competing against yourself, refusing to be satisfied with being better than others when you know you haven't reached your own full potential. Martial arts training creates warriors because it provides both the external challenges—sparring partners, tournaments, tests—and the internal process for honest self-assessment.

You are the ninja on the mountain. Look for the opportunity to train against yourself, to see how much better you can become. As you explore your capabilities the experience will accumulate positive emotional memories, which develop your psychological flexibility and adaptive capacity, allowing you to recover quickly from setbacks and navigate adversity. Each success in overcoming challenges—whether mastering complex techniques or competing in sparring matches—reinforces feelings of accomplishment, persistence, and self-discipline, which cumulatively contribute to the development of resilience. Your ninja on the mountain story will enhance your ability to handle life's big challenges, not just in the ring, but common conflicts and everyday struggles.

Common Ground

Polished warriors share certain qualities that martial arts training develops systematically:

Discipline: The daily commitment to show up and train, regardless of how you feel. Discipline is doing what needs to be done when it needs to be done, whether convenient or not.

Dedication: Staying committed to the path even when progress feels slow, when you're injured, when life gets in the way. Dedication means you don't quit when it gets hard—you recommit.

Self-Respect: Understanding your worth and refusing to compromise your values. Self-respect means treating your body, mind, and spirit with the care they deserve. It means not accepting mediocrity from yourself.

Integrity: Alignment between what you say and what you do. Warriors are honest with themselves about their capabilities and limitations. In fighting, truth is the obstacle to overcome for success—with truth, there is progress; without it, wasted time and mistakes.

Work Ethic: The willingness to put in the hours, the sweat, the pain. Warriors understand that there are no shortcuts. Choosing the short cut always ends up being the longest road. The basics cannot be skipped and until they are mastered your goals will always remain out of reach.

Focus: The ability to concentrate completely on the task at hand. Focus means being present in the moment, facing reality and the truth of what is happening with and around you.

Perseverance: Continuing when every instinct tells you to stop. Perseverance is the refusal to quit, even when quitting would be easier, more comfortable, more socially acceptable.

These aren't abstract virtues. They're trainable skills that martial arts systematically develops through repetition, testing, and the constant cycle of challenge and growth.

Love is Strength

The martial arts are a practice in love—love of life and all one holds dear. The martial arts provide the ability to defend oneself and preserve family and friends.

Love for others is not weakness disguised as strength. Love is the strongest possible motivation: training with the aim to be able to defend cherished ones. This motivation has kept warriors fighting and training through countless dreary days, through injuries, through doubt – across time immemorial.

Imagine if every hero and great warrior had listened to those around them who told them, "It cannot be done." Greater warriors have tried and failed, they'll say. You cannot do it, give up. Ignore this, instead listen to those who love and support you. Love is not jealous of your personal betterment and advancement. Love wants you to succeed.

Every task at its infancy seems impossibly uphill. An insurmountable challenge. Negativity is no friend and neither are those that peddle in it. Shake off the naysayers and carry on.

Love is a powerful motivator. Being in love with the martial arts has brought me amazing experiences and outstanding people. But more importantly, the love of what and who you're protecting transforms training from a hobby into a calling. With greater capacity to protect, you may love even stronger, as the fear of loss is greatly diminished. Embrace your love of others and turn it into your most powerful motivator to train.

When you understand what you're fighting for, the sacrifices don't feel like sacrifices. They feel like investments in the safety and well being of everything that matters.

Strategy and Patience: The Warrior's Mind

Warriors don't win through aggression alone. They win through strategy and patience, like asymmetric warfare where the smaller force defeats the larger through superior tactics and adaptability.

Studying military tactics from any era will bring enlightenment to the fight game. The principles of combat are transferable from one genre to the next. There is a mental technique that fundamentally changed the way I approached decision-making of any sort. It came from an Air Force colonel who could beat anyone in the sky in under forty seconds.

Let me show you how it works.

The OODA Loop: Colonel John Boyd's Gift to Warriors;

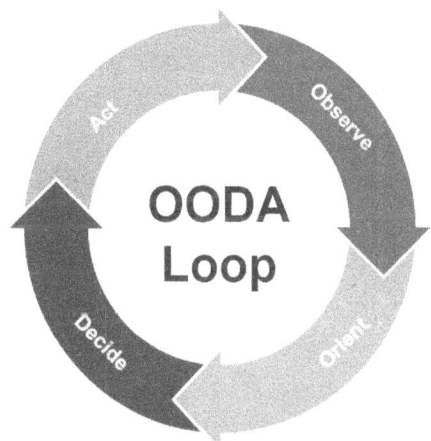

Picture this scenario:

You're in the ring. Your opponent circles left, then suddenly shifts right. His shoulder drops slightly—is he setting up a hook or faking to draw your guard down? His weight transfers to his front foot. You have maybe half a second to decide: step back, counter with a jab, slip inside, or hold position?

The untrained fighter sees the shoulder drop and reacts instinctively, walking straight into the trap. His guard goes up for the hook that never comes, and the real attack—a low kick—sweeps his legs. He's on the canvas wondering what happened. He saw the same thing you saw. Why did you win and he lost?

The answer isn't strictly in speed, nor power. It's basic: you completed your decision-making cycle faster than he completed his. You observed the same information, but you processed it more efficiently and acted while he was still thinking. This same OODA Loop can be it utilized everywhere in your daily life— yes, in combat, but also in business negotiations, relationships, even traffic situations.

The man who discovered this principle was Colonel John Boyd.

Boyd was a United States Air Force fighter pilot who revolutionized modern combat theory. In the 1950s and '60s, he earned the nickname "40-Second Boyd" because he could defeat any opponent in air combat maneuvering in less than forty seconds. Forty seconds. Think about that. Experienced pilots with thousands of flight hours would face Boyd, confident in their skills, and within forty seconds they'd be comprehensively beaten. Every single time.

But Boyd's greatest contribution wasn't his skill in the cockpit—it was his understanding of how decisions are made under pressure. He realized that combat, whether in the air or on the ground, isn't primarily about weapons or physical capability. It's about who can make better decisions faster. The person who can cycle through their decision-making process more rapidly than their opponent doesn't just have an advantage—they dominate completely.

Boyd called this decision-making process the OODA Loop: Observe, Orient, Decide, Act.

Now let me show you how this works by walking you through that fight scenario again—but this time, we'll slow it down and see what's actually happening in each phase.

Your opponent circles left, then shifts right. Activate **the Observe phase.** You're gathering raw data through your senses. You see his footwork change. You notice his shoulder drop. You register the weight transfer to his front foot. You're also observing his breathing pattern, his eye focus, even the slight tension in his jaw. Many fighters stop here—they see only the obvious surface action. But observation is more than just watching. It's active data collection across multiple channels simultaneously. The more complete your observation, the better your next phase will be.

But observation alone means nothing without the Orient phase.

Orient means taking that raw data and filtering it through your knowledge, experience, and cultural understanding to determine what it actually means. It is not a conscious process—it happens in milliseconds. Your brain is running pattern recognition: "I've seen this setup before. When opponents shift right after circling left, they're usually setting up power shots from their dominant side. But his shoulder drop is exaggerated—too obvious. That's often a feint. And the weight transfer is incomplete—if he was really committed to a hook, his whole body would rotate more. This feels like a fake to draw my guard up so he can attack low."

All of that analysis happens faster than you can articulate it. The Orient phase is why experience matters so much in fighting. A beginner sees the shoulder drop and thinks "punch incoming." An experienced fighter sees the same shoulder drop and thinks "fake, watch for the real attack." Same observation. Completely different orientation. Different orientation leads to different decisions.

Which brings us to the Decide phase.

Based on your observation (shoulder drop, weight transfer, footwork) and your orientation (this is probably a fake), you must now choose your response. Do you: step back to create distance? Counter-strike to interrupt whatever he's planning? Slip inside to smother the technique? Or check low to defend against the kick you suspect is coming?

Now, the critical moment. You've got all the data. You've interpreted it. Now you must commit to an action. The decision doesn't have to be perfect—it just has to be made. Hesitation kills. The fighter who observes correctly, orients accurately, but freezes at the decision point loses to the fighter who makes a slightly wrong decision but commits to it immediately.

You decide: check low, then counter immediately.

Now comes Act—the only phase your opponent can actually see.

Your shin comes up to block the low kick you anticipated. His kick slams into your check—exactly as you predicted. Before he can recover, you're already acting on the next cycle: you've observed his balance is compromised, oriented to the fact that he's vulnerable for the next half-second, decided to counter with a straight right, and now you're throwing it. Your fist connects clean.

From your opponent's perspective, here's what just happened:

He set up what he thought was a clever feint. He executed it well. But somehow you weren't fooled. Worse, you were already countering before he could reset. It feels like you read his mind. Like you're impossibly fast. But you're not reading his mind, and you're not faster than him physically. You're simply completing your OODA Loop faster than he completes his.

While he was still observing the results of his fake (did it work?), you had already oriented (it didn't work, I blocked it), decided (counter now while he's off-balance), and acted (thrown the punch). You lapped him. You completed an entire decision cycle while he was still stuck in his first one.

And here's where it gets devastating.

Now your opponent is behind. He has to observe that your punch is coming, orient to this new threat, decide how to defend, and act on that decision. But you're not waiting. You're already into your next OODA Loop: observing how he reacts to your punch, orienting to his defensive pattern, deciding on your next strike, and acting. You're making decisions faster than he can respond to them. You're inside his decision-making cycle, which means you're controlling the entire fight.

Boyd discovered: **the person who consistently completes their OODA Loop faster doesn't just win—they create a psychological cascade in their opponent.** The opponent becomes reactive, defensive, confused. They lose the initiative completely. They're always responding to your last move instead of executing their own strategy. And the more behind they fall, the more desperate and sloppy their decisions become, which makes them even easier to beat.

Now let's see this same principle operating outside the ring.

Imagine you're in a business negotiation. The other party makes an offer. Most people observe the offer (the numbers, the terms), but they orient poorly—they react emotionally, feeling insulted or excited without analyzing the strategic position. Or they orient correctly but freeze at the decision phase, asking for time to "think about it" while their opponent moves forward with additional pressure tactics.

But if you understand the OODA Loop, you observe the offer completely (not just the headline number but the body language, timing, and what's not being said). You orient strategically (what does this offer reveal about their position? What pressure are they under? What are they really after?). You decide quickly (counter with specific modifications, or accept, or walk away). And you act decisively—no hemming and hawing, no visible uncertainty.

You've completed your loop. Now they have to observe your response, orient to this new situation, decide how to counter, and act. But you're not waiting. You're already observing their reaction to your counter, orienting to what it reveals about their priorities, deciding on your next move, and acting. You're inside their decision cycle, which means you control the negotiation.

The same pattern appears in everyday conflicts.

Your partner starts an argument. Insecure people observe the words being said and immediately react emotionally—that's skipping the Orient and Decide phases entirely and going straight to an Act that's purely emotional. The fight escalates because neither person is actually thinking. But if you observe what's being said, orient to what's really driving this (is this about the dishes or about feeling unappreciated?), decide on a strategic response (acknowledge the real issue, not just the surface complaint), and act accordingly—you short-circuit the whole conflict. You've operated at a higher level of decision-making, and the entire dynamic changes.

Here's what makes the OODA Loop so powerful: it's fractal.

It operates at every timescale. In a fistfight, you're running through OODA Loops every few seconds. In a business strategy, you might run through one over weeks or months. But the principle is identical: observe accurately, orient strategically, decide quickly, act decisively, then immediately start the next cycle.

And here's the key insight that separates masters from

amateurs: **you can train each phase independently to speed up your entire loop.**

Improve your Observe phase by becoming more aware, more present, more attuned to subtle signals. Martial arts training does this systematically—you learn to see feints, read body language, detect weight shifts. This observation skill transfers everywhere. You start noticing micro-expressions in negotiations, subtext in conversations, patterns in market behavior.

Strengthen your Orient phase by studying strategy, learning from experience, and deliberately analyzing situations instead of reacting instinctively. Every time you spar and then review what happened—what worked, what failed, why—you're building better orientation. You're creating a mental database of patterns that lets you interpret new situations more accurately and more quickly.

Accelerate your Decide phase by practicing decision-making under pressure and why hard sparring is invaluable. You can't afford to freeze. You must choose: defend, counter, evade, advance. None of these choices is perfect, but doing something beats doing nothing. The more you practice making imperfect decisions quickly, the better your decisions become and the faster you make them.

Refine your Act phase through technical mastery and conditioning. When you decide to throw a combination, your body needs to execute it without conscious thought. It's why we drill techniques thousands of times—so that when your decision arrives, your action follows instantly with precision. No hesitation between decision and execution. The technique fires the moment you will it.

Train all four phases, and something remarkable happens.

Your OODA Loop accelerates. You observe more, orient better, decide faster, and act more decisively than your opponents.

In a fight, this feels like precognition. In business, it feels like strategic genius. In relationships, it feels like emotional intelligence. But it's not magic—it's a trainable skill.

And here's the final insight that makes this truly dangerous:

Once you understand the OODA Loop, you can deliberately disrupt your opponent's cycle. You can feed them false information during their Observe phase—feints, misdirection, lies. You can confuse their Orient phase by doing unexpected things that don't fit their mental models. You can paralyze their Decide phase by presenting too many options or creating time pressure. And you can interrupt their Act phase by striking first or changing the environment while they're mid-action.

Meanwhile, you're protecting your own loop. You're observing from multiple sources so you can't be easily deceived. You're orienting from principles rather than assumptions so you adapt quickly to the unexpected. You're deciding based on strategy rather than emotion so you don't get baited into bad choices. And you're acting with commitment so you can't be easily countered mid-execution.

Colonel Boyd was unbeatable and why experienced fighters dismantle beginners even when the beginners are younger, stronger, and faster. This exact method why some business leaders seem to operate three moves ahead of their competition. They're not necessarily smarter, and they're definitely not gifted with supernatural intuition. Consciously or unconsciously, they've simply mastered the OODA Loop—and they're running it faster than everyone else.

The warrior path teaches this through direct, unforgiving experience.

Every sparring session is OODA Loop training. Every tournament is a test of how fast you can cycle through decisions under maximum pressure. Every technique you drill is building the automatic responses that speed up your Act phase. Every moment you spend analyzing your performance is strengthening your Orient phase.

And once you've internalized this framework from martial arts training, you carry it everywhere. The job interview becomes an OODA Loop competition. The difficult conversation with your teenager becomes strategic decision-making. The crisis at work becomes an opportunity to observe, orient, decide, and act while others are still panicking.

Immense training depth across the entire human canvas is what separates warriors from everyone else. Not just the ability to fight, but the ability to think clearly under pressure, make decisions rapidly, and act decisively while others hesitate. The OODA Loop is the mental weapon that makes everything else possible.

Master it, and you don't just become a better fighter. You become dangerous in every arena of life.

More Sweat in Practice, Less Blood in War

This ancient wisdom holds true: the more you suffer in training, the less you suffer in real conflict.

Train harder than you think you can. Always push yourself to new challenges and new achievements, and you will astonish your enemies and yourself.

Train in the mirror and record it on camera. Watch the footage and be your own worst critic. Always strive to train as hard as you know you can – not just good enough – to your maximum!

Train to impress yourself, and you will never be a mediocre fighter, because everyone else is training only to the level of their current sparring partners. Train to never let yourself down. Invest in yourself, you will repay the highest dividends.

Fighting is hard, and the physical exhaustion can happen quickly. Getting overwhelmed from lack of preparation has been the most humbling and most frustrating. Ask yourself honestly, are you actually well prepared? Are you doing the minimum, is your effort lacking in any way? Did you put your entire being into your mission readiness? You will not get a chance to do this challenge again, so give it your all from the very first day that you set a goal.

The ninja on the mountain principle applies here: don't measure yourself against others. Measure yourself against your potential. The gap between where you are and where you could be—that's your real opponent.

Two thousand years ago, when Caesar set out to conquer England by water, after landing ashore, he found himself face to face with his own soldiers preparing to retreat, swallowed by their own fears—some very real and valid ones at that.

In response, Julius Caesar famously ordered: "If you want to take this island, burn the boats!"

Caesar knew about the art of war. He ordered all the ships burned. This was a powerful message to his enemies, but an even more powerful one to his own men. With no ability to retreat, his army was now 100% committed to doing whatever it took to succeed. And if they didn't, it certainly would not be for lack of effort or courage. If they didn't, they would be dead.

Here marks the depth at which you must be committed to winning. A warrior has no qualms with advancing while giving up the ability to retreat.

In 1775, Patrick Henry, an American founding father, proclaimed: "Give me liberty, or give me death." A timeless creed for any warrior for freedom. It means we will advance our position and meet our goals, and there will be no other option.

Warriors understand that some things are worth more than survival. Some causes demand total commitment. When you truly commit—when you burn the boats—you discover reserves of strength and determination you didn't know you possessed.

Warrior's Test

I lived my first burn the boats event on a cold winter evening outside a nightclub in Abbotsford, British Columbia. It was during a spat of heightened gang violence around the area. We had had some shootings and stabbings too, one of which the victims entrails were pulled out of his stomach by the attacker and left on the pavement. It was one of two murders around the club over the past few months, and a gruesome one at that.

I was working as a doorman, walking a woman to her car around closing. Four men approached me—the same four we had thrown out earlier that evening. They were back for revenge.

No backup. The side of the building had no doors, no cameras, no way to be seen. They surrounded me in an arc to my front.

In that moment, I accepted I was going to lose badly. Four against one, ambushed, isolated—the math wasn't in my favor. But I also decided: I was going to get one hard strike in on each of them first.

I started by hitting the one who moved closest, then immediately pivoted to the man moving to me on the right. By the time I hit the third person in quick succession, they collectively looked at each other and decided to back away.

It was a good thing. I shattered my right fist on the top of the skull of the third person as he was ducking. My power hand was out of commission. I have a boxer's fracture with deformed knuckles to this day from that altercation. Luckily they were looking for an easy win and were not fully committed to the fight. Had they pressed further they would have known I was injured.

What did I learn?

First, commitment is key. The moment I accepted the fight and committed fully—no retreat, no hesitation—the energy shifted. They felt it.

Second, action beats reaction. I didn't wait for them to coordinate. I attacked first, creating chaos in their plan. I wasn't intimidated in the least, and that surprised them.

Third, violence has consequences. My hand serves as a permanent reminder that even when you "win," real violence costs you something.

Fourth, training works. Breathing, footwork, pivots, weight transfers, targeting, distance. Every technique I used that night had been drilled hundreds of times. No thought, just action. My body knew what to do when my mind didn't have time to think.

That's what it means to be a warrior: accepting the fight that's coming, committing fully, acting decisively, and understanding that even victory leaves scars.

Daily Grind

"Life is about fighting. You are going to have to fight every day of your lifetime."—Renzo Gracie, 2011

Gracie is right, but not in the way most people think. Most days, you won't fight with your fists. You'll fight against laziness, fear, doubt, complacency, mediocrity. You'll fight to get out of bed when you're exhausted. You'll fight to stay disciplined when no one's watching. You'll fight to keep your word when breaking it would be easier. A majority of the time, the battle is with yourself.

The warrior mindset isn't about violence. It's about refusing to quit when life gets hard.

The challenge of becoming this person is a daily struggle you must take up with fervor. There is no time to lose, and the competition is fierce—not against others, but against your own potential left unrealized.

Combat martial arts provide participants with frequent opportunities to face and overcome challenges. Each success reinforces feelings of accomplishment, persistence, and self-discipline. These positive experiences accumulate over time, creating psychological flexibility and adaptive capacity.

Warriors aren't born. They're forged through the daily decision to show up, train hard, face truth, and refuse to quit.

Service & Sacrifice

The warrior's true purpose centers not on personal glory, but service. Not dominance, but protection. Not violence for its own sake, but the capability and willingness to stand between those you love and whatever threatens them.

Martial arts training creates warriors by systematically developing the characteristics—discipline, dedication, integrity, focus, perseverance—and the mindset—adaptability, honesty, strategic thinking, resilience—that allow you to rise to every occasion.

You manifest the warrior by training against yourself, measuring your progress against your potential rather than against others. You manifest the warrior by committing fully, burning the boats, refusing the option of retreat. You manifest the warrior by loving what you're fighting for deeply enough that the sacrifices feel like investments.

Fall seven times, get up eight (nana korobi ya oki 七転び八起き). Japanese Proverb

A warrior rises to the occasion. Over and over again.

The warrior path isn't easy. If it were, everyone would walk it. But those who do find that the person they become through the journey is worth every drop of sweat, every moment of doubt overcome, every time they stood up after being knocked down.

Knocked down seven times, stand up eight.

That's what warriors do.

Now you know what a warrior is and how martial arts

training creates one. We need to examine our human emotions and how to get them working for us by mastering them.

CHAPTER 4 – MASTER EMOTIONS

"In a very real sense we have two minds, one that thinks and one that feels."—Daniel Goleman, Emotional Intelligence. 1995

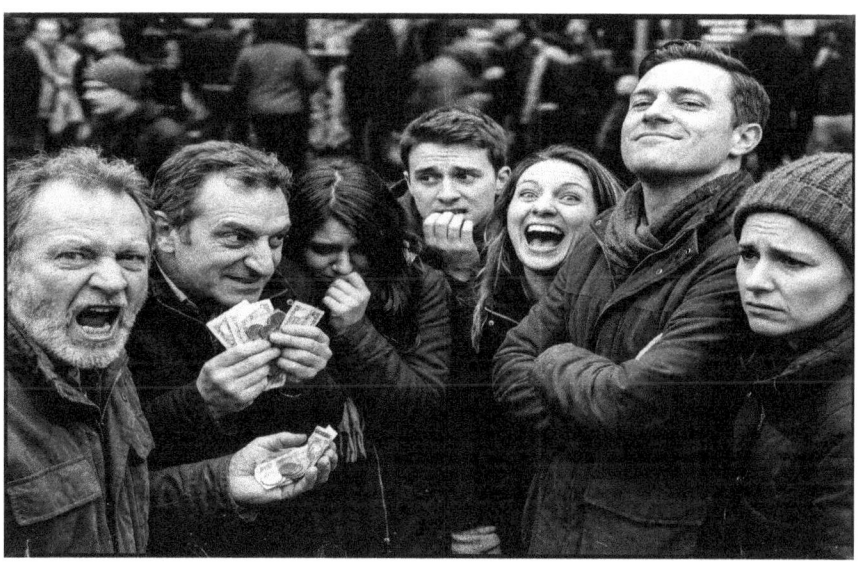

Invisible Opponent

There is an opponent you face in every fight that most warriors never recognize. It's not the person across from you in the ring. It's not the opponent you've studied and prepared for. It's the storm inside your own chest. Your emotions are the most dangerous adversary you'll ever face because they're with you in every moment, influencing every decision, coloring every perception, driving every action.

Fear. Anger. Pride. Shame. Joy. Desperation. These forces move through you like weather patterns, sometimes gentle breezes, sometimes hurricanes that tear everything apart. The untrained brawler is a slave to these forces. They react. They get angry and throw wild punches. They get scared and freeze. They get overconfident and drop their guard. Every emotion pulls the strings and they dance like puppets.

The warrior learns to feel everything and be controlled by nothing. One doesn't suppress emotions or pretend they don't exist. That's a fool's game that leads to explosions at the worst possible moments. No, this is about developing a relationship with your emotional state where you acknowledge what you're feeling, understand why you're feeling it, and choose consciously how to respond.

"The ultimate aim of martial arts is not having to use them; it is to perfect the self and control one's emotions so that conflict becomes unnecessary." —Bruce Lee, 1968

Emotional mastery is the difference between a good fighter and a great one. It's the difference between a successful person and someone who constantly sabotages themselves. It's the difference between shallow relationships and deep connections. Your technical skills only take you so far. Your emotional control determines how far you actually go.

Let's get real about what's happening when emotions hit. Your body is an ancient survival machine that hasn't gotten the software update that we're not being chased by saber-toothed tigers anymore. Intense fear and anger can both trigger what is known as the "fight or flight" response. Some people freeze in this condition, others turn and run for the hills when the feeling hits. But warriors must train to fight with it and through it.

Dance with Fear

Fear is married to the fight-or-flight response, and it's kept the human species alive since our ancient past. But here's the problem: in a modern context, this response often makes things worse. Fear triggers anger and that triggers the response. You get angry at your business partner and your body prepares you to punch them, when what you actually need is clear thinking and concise communication. You get nervous before a competition and your body locks up, when what you need is fluid movement and quick reactions. Our primitive animal systems that are instinctively induced can take years of practice to master.

The martial artist trains to override these automatic responses. Not by eliminating them—you can't, they're hardwired—but by recognizing them early and choosing a different path. Hence why we drill techniques ten thousand times. We're not just training muscles, we're rewiring neural pathways so that when the amygdala fires, when the stress hormones flood, when the thinking brain goes offline—the trained response kicks in automatically.

In the ring, this looks like staying calm under pressure. In business, this looks like making rational decisions when everyone else is panicking. In relationships, this looks like responding thoughtfully instead of reacting defensively.

Fear is your constant companion as a warrior. Anyone who tells you they feel no fear is either lying or dangerously disconnected from reality. Fear is information. It tells you that something important needs your attention, that there's risk, that you need to be alert. The question is not whether you feel fear, but what you do with it.

There are two types of fear in combat. The first is healthy **respect**—the awareness that your opponent is dangerous, that mistakes have consequences, that you need to be sharp. This fear keeps you alive. It makes you train harder. It keeps your guard up. Using fear as an ally.

The second type is **paralyzing** terror—the fear that makes you hesitate, that makes you doubt yourself, that makes you want to run. This fear gets you hurt. It makes you tentative. It makes you predictable. Here is: Fear as an enemy.

The difference between these two types of fear is where you place your attention. If your attention is on the threat—on how much bigger your opponent is, on how badly this could go, on all the ways you might lose—that's paralyzing fear. If your attention is on your response—on your technique, on your breathing, on the opportunities you're creating—that's healthy respect.

You control fear by controlling attention. Where your eyes go, your mind follows. Where your mind goes, your body follows. In the ring, you train yourself to focus on what you can do, not what might happen to you. This same principle applies everywhere. The business presentation that terrifies you becomes manageable when you focus on delivering value rather than being judged. The difficult conversation becomes possible when you focus on understanding rather than defending. Perspective is everything.

Fear never goes away. You just get better at dancing with it.

Anger: Fuel or Fire

> *"When anger arises, think of the consequences."*
> *Confucius. 462BCE*

Anger is a gift and a curse. It can make you powerful or it can make you stupid. The difference is control.

Uncontrolled anger is the amateur's mistake. They get hit, they get mad, they rush forward throwing wild combinations with their chin up and their guard down. They're easy to read, easy to counter, easy to finish. Their anger made them predictable. It blinded them to danger. It robbed them of technique.

Every experienced fighter has beaten someone bigger and stronger simply by making them angry and waiting for them to make mistakes.

Controlled anger is different. A righteous focused anger. An anger that you consciously harness as fuel without letting it drive the car. You feel it, you acknowledge it, you use the energy it provides—but you don't let it make decisions. Your technique stays tight. Your vision stays clear. Your strategy stays intact. You're just executing that strategy with more intensity.

In competition, this looks like the fighter who gets hit with a cheap shot and instead of losing composure, tightens up their defense and starts systematically breaking down their opponent with precision. The anger is there—you can see it in their eyes—but it's serving them, not controlling them.

In business, this is the entrepreneur who gets screwed over by a partner and instead of seeking petty revenge, channels that anger into building something better. The anger motivated them, but wisdom guided them.

In relationships, this is the person who feels hurt and angry but takes a breath before speaking, who expresses their feelings without attacking, who uses the emotional energy to create change rather than damage.

Here's the key: Anger makes you aggressive. Anger makes you strong but it makes you stupid. The warrior's task is to keep the strength and reject the stupidity. Feel the anger. Let it energize you. Then put your thinking brain back in charge and execute your strategy with that extra horsepower behind it.

Pride

We have all heard that pride comes before the fall. Pride is the emotion that sneaks up on successful warriors and destroys them. You've trained for years. You've won fights. You've earned respect. You start to believe your own legend. You stop training as hard because you figure you're already good enough. You underestimate opponents. You take unnecessary risks because you need to prove something.

Then someone humbles you, and if you're lucky, you learn from it. If you're not lucky, you make excuses and blame others and never grow past that defeat; or possibly much worse.

Anyone paying attention has seen more potential champions destroyed by pride than by any opponent. Pride is the voice that says "I don't need to drill that basic technique, I'm beyond that." Pride is what makes you refuse to tap when you're caught in a submission, so you get injured. Pride is what makes you challenge people unnecessarily to prove you're tough. Pride is exhausting and expensive.

Humility

Humility is the antidote. Not false humility where you pretend to be less capable than you are—that's just pride in disguise. Real humility is accurate self-assessment. You know your strengths and you leverage them. You know your weaknesses and you work on them. You respect every opponent because you understand that on any given day, anyone can win.

The truly dangerous fighters are the humble ones. They have nothing to prove. They don't need to showboat. They don't need to talk. They just show up, do the work, and let the results speak. In business, these are the quiet professionals who outwork everyone without needing recognition. In relationships, these are the people who can admit when they're wrong and apologize without their ego collapsing.

Pride says "I'm the best." Humility says "I'm working to be better than I was yesterday." One leads to stagnation. The other leads to continuous growth.

Two Advantageous Emotions

Here's something other martial arts books won't tell you: Joy and love are tactical advantages.

The fighter who genuinely loves the process—who enjoys training, who finds their flow in sparring, who appreciates the journey—will always outlast the fighter who's just grinding through suffering. Enjoyment is sustainable. Misery is not. If you hate training, you'll quit eventually. If you love it, you'll do it for life. Having an instructor you admire and partners who inject love and joy in your sessions will promote the desired atmosphere keeping you engaged long term.

I've watched students with less natural talent surpass more gifted athletes simply because they loved the art. They showed up more consistently. They trained with more enthusiasm. They approached every session as an opportunity rather than an obligation. That attitude compounds over years into mastery.

The same applies to business. The entrepreneur who loves solving problems will persist through failures that would break someone who's just chasing money. The person who loves learning will continuously improve while others stagnate.

And in relationships? Love is the whole game. The person who approaches relationships with genuine care and joy, who loves supporting their partner's growth, who finds happiness in connection—they build something that lasts. The person who sees relationships as transactions or obligations creates hollow connections that eventually collapse.

Joy is an amazing weapon in competition, and can be a game changer in anything you set out to do. The fighter who's genuinely having fun is relaxed, creative, unpredictable. They're not tight with tension. They're not rigid with fear. They flow. They adapt. They see opportunities that the stressed fighter misses. Muhammad Ali made fighting look like dancing because he enjoyed it. That enjoyment was part of what made him great. Finding joy in a fight is liberating and fun, and it can really confuse those opponents who are running on anger or fear as their primary operating system.

Find what you love about this journey and protect it. Let it fuel you when discipline wavers. Let it sustain you through the hard years. Let it remind you why you started when you're tempted to quit. And try to have some fun while you are doing it.

Shame and Guilt

There are some other emotions that are perhaps on the fringe of our radar as emotions that need mastery. Shame and guilt are the heavy chains that so many people drag through life without even realizing it. Shame says "I am bad." Guilt says "I did something bad." Both will destroy your performance if you don't address them.

In the ring, shame shows up as the voice that says you're not good enough, you don't belong here, everyone's going to see you're a fraud. It makes you hesitant. It makes you apologize for taking up space. It makes you quit before you even start because you're convinced you'll fail anyway.

Guilt shows up as the weight of past mistakes. The time you froze in a fight. The time you let your team down. The time you quit when it got hard. These memories replay in your mind and convince you that you'll fail again.

Here's the truth: Everyone has moments they're ashamed of. Everyone has made mistakes. The warrior acknowledges these moments, learns from them, and moves forward. Shame and guilt are only useful if they teach you something. If they're just background noise making you feel bad, they're useless weight.

The way out is through acceptance and action. Accept that you're human, that you've made mistakes, that you'll make more. Then take action to be better today than you were yesterday. Replace the shame narrative ("I'm not good enough") with an accurate assessment ("I'm learning and improving").

Replace guilt ("I failed before") with commitment ("I'll do better this time").

In business, shame and guilt make you scared to take risks, scared to put yourself out there, scared to claim your worth. In relationships, they make you tolerate mistreatment because you don't believe you deserve better.

Cut those chains. You're carrying enough weight with your actual responsibilities. Don't add imaginary weight just because your brain likes to torture you. It does not matter what you did, you cannot change that. It only matters what you do, because that is still happening.

Emotional Contagion: Reading the Room

Here's something powerful that poorly trained fighters don't consciously understand: Emotions are contagious. Your emotional state affects everyone around you, and their emotional state affects you. In a fight, if you're calm and confident, your opponent feels it and often starts doubting themselves. If you're nervous and unsure, they feel that too and gain confidence.

Recognize emotional contagion in action. Harnessing and controlling it gives you a massive advantage. You can consciously project the emotional state that serves your strategy. You want your opponent anxious? Show them calm confidence and make them question why you're so relaxed. You want them overconfident? Show them nervousness and let them rush in recklessly.

But this cuts both ways. If you're not careful, you'll absorb the emotions of people around you. You're backstage before a fight and everyone's freaking out, suddenly you're anxious even though you were calm a minute ago. You're in a business meeting and everyone's angry, suddenly you're angry too without even knowing why.

The martial artist trains to maintain their center regardless of the emotional weather around them. You feel the emotions, you notice them, but you don't let them pull you off your foundation. Advanced work, yes, but it's critical.

In relationships, emotional contagion is why you need to be conscious of the energy you bring home. If you walk in stressed and angry, you'll spread that through your household. If you walk in with love and presence, you'll create that atmosphere instead. You're not responsible for other people's emotions, but you are responsible for the emotional weather you create.

The take-away; Read the room. Notice the emotional undercurrents. Choose consciously what emotional state you want to embody and project. Don't just react to whatever emotion is most prominent in your environment.

The Pause: a Momentary Calm

Between stimulus and response, there is a space. In that space lies your power to choose and where emotional mastery lives. In the OODA loop it is the split second between Orient and Decide. It happens as something has been observed and you orient your thinking to the situation and begin processing. You quickly gather information and prepare to make a deliberate decision. It is this split second of processing that is **the pause,** the eye of the storm.

Let's examine this space in time closer. Someone insults you. There's a moment—maybe just a second—before you respond. The untrained person reacts immediately. Insult triggers anger triggers verbal attack or physical violence. It cascades. It's automatic. It's predictable. It's weak.

The trained warrior capitalizes on this space or pause. They feel the anger rising. They recognize the impulse to strike back. And in that moment, they choose. Maybe they laugh loudly and defuse. Maybe they respond with calm confidence that makes the insult powerless. Maybe they ignore it completely.

Maybe they do respond with violence, but it's a choice, not a reaction. The control is what matters.

This pause is what you're training every time you drill techniques under pressure. You're expanding that space between stimulus and response. You're creating room for choice. The beginner gets hit and immediately reacts with tension and panic. The advanced practitioner gets hit and has enough space to stay relaxed, assess, and respond strategically. In a real fight it is common for combatants to say time slowed down, every move was in slow motion. These are the moments we want to create.

In business, the pause is what separates leaders from followers. Bad news hits. The follower panics immediately. The leader takes a breath, assesses, then responds with a plan. That pause—even if it's just three seconds—makes all the difference in the world.

In relationships, the pause is what saves marriages. Your partner says something that hurts. The pause is where you choose between defensive attack and vulnerable honesty. Between escalation and resolution. Between reaction and response.

Train the pause. Literally practice it. When you're drilling and something doesn't go as planned, pause before reacting. When you're in conversation and you feel emotion rising, pause before speaking. Make the pause automatic. Make it your default response to any strong emotion.

Meditate for Emotional Mastery

You can't master your emotions without training them directly, and that training is meditation. Not some mystical woo-woo nonsense—practical, tactical meditation that builds your capacity to observe your inner experience without being overwhelmed by it.

Sit. Breathe. Notice your thoughts and feelings as they

arise. Don't fight them. Don't judge them. Just notice them. "Oh, there's anxiety." "Oh, there's anger." "Oh, there's that story about how I'm not good enough." Notice it like you'd notice clouds passing in the sky. They come, they go, you remain.

The same skill serves you in the ring. Opponent throws a combination. You notice it without panicking. You respond. Emotion rises in your chest. You notice it without panicking. You respond.

Most people are so identified with their emotions that they think they *are* their emotions. "I'm angry" becomes their entire identity in that moment. Meditation teaches you that you're not your emotions. You're the awareness that observes emotions. That shift in perspective is freedom.

Start with five minutes a day. Just sit and breathe and notice. you will wander—that's fine, that's what minds do. Notice it wandering and gently bring attention back to breath. You're not trying to stop thoughts or achieve some blissed-out state. You're training the muscle of attention. You're creating space between you and your experience.

Do this consistently and you'll notice that emotions have less power over you. You'll feel anger and be able to act rationally. You'll feel fear and be able to move forward anyway. You'll feel joy without clinging to it. You'll feel pain without being destroyed by it.

"The mind is everything. What you think you become." Buddha. 598BCE

The mind and where you focus attention will set your emotional starting point for every decision, every action. Using meditation to recenter your mind to clear irrational thought is essential on a daily basis. Every great warrior tradition includes some form of meditation practice. There's a reason for that. It works.

Emotional Intelligence for Fighters

In competition, emotional intelligence is what separates champions from also-rans. Technical skill gets you in the door. Emotional mastery determines how far you go.

The emotionally intelligent fighter reads their opponent's emotional state and exploits it. They see the opponent getting frustrated and they make it worse with feints and angles that increase that frustration. They see the opponent getting overconfident and they let them overextend so they can counter. They see the opponent getting tired and demoralized and they press the attack to break their will.

Simultaneously, they manage their own emotional state. They stay calm when they're winning so they don't get cocky. They stay composed when they're losing so they can find a path back. They feel everything—the fatigue, the pain, the fear, the exhilaration—but none of it controls them.

The fighter with superior emotional intelligence will often beat the fighter with superior technical skill because they're playing a different game. The technical fighter is focused on techniques. The emotionally intelligent fighter is focused on breaking the opponent's will, on creating doubt, on manufacturing psychological advantages that create openings for techniques.

Fighters must be able to navigate emotional maturity throughout their lives, and know how to keep the fights where they belong – in the ring or as the last resort. But emotions spikes can strike like lightning, unexpected, and catch us by surprise in everyday situations. These are other training opportunities to test our skills for control of our emotions.

Emotional Intelligence in Business

In business, emotional intelligence is the difference between someone who's technically competent and someone who leads. The emotionally intelligent business person reads the room in negotiations. They understand what motivates their team members individually. They know when to push and when to support. They can deliver bad news in a way that maintains morale. They can celebrate wins without creating complacency.

They also manage their own emotional state through the chaos of entrepreneurship. They feel the fear of financial uncertainty but make rational decisions anyway. They feel the anger of betrayal or unfairness but respond strategically rather than impulsively. They feel the joy of success but stay hungry for more growth.

The business leader who lacks emotional intelligence might have great ideas and strong technical skills, but they'll struggle to build teams, maintain relationships, and navigate the human complexity of organizations. They'll wonder why people don't follow them, not realizing that their inability to manage their own emotions or read others is the problem.

Emotional intelligence is learnable. Pay attention to what you're feeling and why. Pay attention to what others are feeling—their body language, their tone, their word choice. Practice responding thoughtfully rather than reactively. Get feedback from people you trust about your emotional impact on others.

Emotional Intelligence in Relationships

In relationships, emotional intelligence is vital. Technical skills don't exist here—there's no technique for loving someone. There's only presence, awareness, empathy, and choice.

The emotionally intelligent partner can feel hurt without attacking. They can express needs without demanding. They can listen to criticism without becoming defensive. They can hold space for their partner's emotions without taking responsibility for fixing them or being destroyed by them.

They understand that their partner's emotions are information, not threats. If their partner is angry, that's data about something that matters to them. If their partner is scared, that's an opportunity to provide security. If their partner is joyful, that's an invitation to celebrate together.

They also take responsibility for their own emotional experience. They don't expect their partner to manage their emotions for them. They don't make their happiness dependent on their partner's behavior. They bring emotional stability to the relationship rather than needing to extract it.

The emotionally unintelligent person in relationships creates constant drama. Everything is a crisis. Every disagreement is an attack. Every emotion is overwhelming. They say things in anger they don't mean. They shut down when they should open up. They demand emotional support while being unable to provide it. They remind me of a squall line (something I have faced as a pilot) or an unstable thunderstorm, with rapid pressure changes, unpredictable lightening and constant instability.

If you want lasting relationships—romantic, friendship, family, business—develop your emotional intelligence. Learn to feel everything and be controlled by nothing. Learn to express yourself clearly without attacking. Learn to listen without defending. Learn to hold complexity without needing to resolve it immediately.

Principles that guide the emotionally masterful warrior:

1. Feel everything. Suppress nothing. Emotions are information. Ignoring them doesn't make them go away, it just makes them leak out in destructive ways. Feel your feelings fully.
2. Be controlled by nothing. Feeling emotions doesn't mean obeying them. You feel fear and advance anyway. You feel anger and stay strategic. You feel joy and stay grounded.
3. The pause is power. Between stimulus and response, choose. Always choose. Never react unconsciously.
4. Your emotional state is your responsibility. No one

"makes" you feel anything. They trigger feelings that exist in you. Own your reactions.

5. Emotions are contagious. Choose wisely. You affect everyone around you. Be conscious of the emotional weather you create.
6. Train the skills. Emotional mastery isn't natural. It's trained. Meditate. Reflect. Practice. Grow.
7. Use emotions as fuel, not as guidance. Anger can energize you, but don't let it drive strategy. Fear can sharpen you, but don't let it paralyze you. Joy can sustain you, but don't let it make you sloppy.
8. Read others without judgment. Notice emotional states in others as tactical information, not as things to fix or criticize.
9. Express clearly without attacking. Say what you feel without making it a weapon. "I feel angry" is different from "You're an asshole."
10. Growth requires discomfort. You will feel things you'd rather not feel. That's the price of emotional development. Pay it.

Martial Arts philosophy and training truly comes together when the warrior is in emotional mastery. The training teaches you to stay present under pressure. The training teaches you to observe without judgment. The spiritual training teaches you to accept reality as it is. All of this culminates in the ability to feel everything life throws at you and respond with wisdom rather than reaction.

The warrior who has mastered their emotions is truly free. Not free from feeling—that would be death. Free to feel fully and choose consciously. Free to love without fear of loss. Free to fight without hatred. Free to lead without ego. Free to connect without dependency.

> "He who controls others may be powerful, but he who has mastered himself is mightier still." Lao Tzu. 600BCE

Now, the last and the final frontier of martial development.

You can have perfect technique, superior conditioning, and brilliant strategy, but if you can't manage your inner experience, you'll always be limited. Your emotions will betray you at critical moments. They'll make you hesitate when you should advance. They'll make you rush when you should wait. They'll make you blind to opportunities and vulnerable to manipulation.

Master your emotions and you master yourself. Master yourself and the world becomes a different place. Not because the world changed, but because you changed. You bring calm to chaos. You bring clarity to confusion. You bring love to places that only knew conflict. You can choose to enjoy every day because you control your feelings, they don't control you.

Emotional Mastery Regime:

Morning:

– Five minutes of meditation. Sit, breathe, observe. Use the (Matt Meditation Method, Ch. 11).

– Set an emotional intention for the day. "Today I choose calm confidence." or "Today I choose joyful presence." On training day "I love being fit!"

Throughout the day:

– Notice the pause before reacting to anything emotional.

– Label emotions as they arise. "I'm feeling anxious." "I'm feeling excited."

– Ask "Is this emotion serving me right now?" If yes, use it. If no, breathe through it.

Training:

– Notice your emotional state during sparring. Are you tense? Frustrated? Flowing?

– Practice staying relaxed when you're losing and humble when you're winning.

– After training, reflect. What emotions showed up? How did you handle them?

Evening:

– Journal about one emotional moment from the day. What

happened? What did you feel?

How did you respond? How do you wish you'd responded?

– Gratitude practice. Name three things you're grateful for. This trains you to notice joy.

<u>Weekly:</u>

– Have one difficult conversation you've been avoiding. Practice emotional clarity without attack.

– Do something that scares you. Train the relationship with fear.

– Do something purely for joy. Train the relationship with pleasure.

Do this for six months and you won't recognize yourself. Do it for five years and you'll be the person others come to when they need wisdom. Do it for life and you'll be free in a way others never experience.

Extreme Emotion

Warriors train for years to avoid needing what I'm about to describe. The goal is emotional mastery, not emotional madness. Control, not chaos. But somewhere deep inside each of us lives an emergency button—a mental switch that summons everything when survival demands it. Brawlers will assume they will probably be able to defend their life if they had to, there is a button, that's all they know. Warriors, preemptively, should unpack and examine it in order to harness it. Understand this button or not, it is in the most dire of circumstances that this emotional whirlwind will arrive and it will be an all-encompassing storm.

The emergency button isn't your first option. Not your second. It's the biggest hammer in the drawer, reserved for the moment when all else has failed and life hangs in the balance.

The Stakes

To engage this way means total commitment. You must be willing to kill. You must be willing to die. These aren't abstractions—they're the actual stakes, with all that entails. Be prepared to say: I will die today if I have to, but that motherfucker is going to pay in blood, and this is a fight to the end. The moment you stop caring whether you live or die, your odds of winning increase substantially. Simultaneously, once they sense your total commitment, your opponent's commitment will waver. Few will follow you to the very end, though many believe they would.

Not panic or flailing. It's channeled fury—laser-focused, lightning-fast, executed with cold temperament and explosive violence. Everything becomes a weapon. Everything becomes a target. Chairs, rocks, dirt, teeth if necessary. Injuries ignored. Broken bones, gunshots, screams, blood—against all inputs, you advance until decisive victory. It is primal, visceral, and void of humanity.

Total domination. Nothing else exists.

The Trap

Here's the danger: rage wears out. If you don't capitalize immediately and dominate quickly, desperation sets in. Then fear. Then fatigue—mental, physical, spiritual. The fighting spirit subsides. The fear of losing becomes real, and it can break your drive entirely.

The calmest person wins because they have staying power. With emotions in check, they make better decisions. Their cardiovascular system doesn't red-line. Their muscles don't pump up uselessly. Their mind stays clear.

Use the emergency button with caution. In chaos, nothing goes to plan. What you risk may exceed what you can calculate.

The Cost

Many war-fighters have pressed this button, some to the point of PTSD. Few talk about it. Anyone who survives life-and-death situations is fundamentally changed. The more "successful" encounters, the more unpredictable the aftermath. Some drown in drugs and alcohol to quiet the storm. Others quit life more directly. Many chase progressively greater risks just to feel that incredible high again.

A close friend is deployed in a hot zone right now—not for ideology, but addiction. The adrenaline switch flipped during his first deployment and never turned off. Now he needs to live between life and death. The civilian world feels empty. Nothing compares to the rush of being shot at. Without combat, he'd need to base-jump exotic canyons until his luck ran out.

The goal is not to eliminate fear, even if you could. You want the alertness it provides without the paralysis or rage. You want sharpness without tunnel vision. You don't want to be a slave to it, crave it, need it, or get lost in it. Fear is just one emotion, it has its place, under control and as a tool, nothing more.

In a Vast Sky

Emotions make you human. Emotional mastery makes you a warrior. Don't confuse the two. Fighting should be a choice, not a reaction. If you are always inexplicably fighting, your emotions are running the show. A warrior picks and plans their battles, a true warrior isn't ambushed by them.

The goal is not to become some stoic robot who feels nothing. The goal is to feel everything fully and respond with wisdom. To cry when crying serves you. To laugh when laughing serves you. To get angry when anger serves you. To feel love without clinging to it. To feel fear without being paralyzed by it.

You are not your emotions. You are the sky. Emotions are weather. Sometimes sunny, sometimes stormy, always changing. The sky doesn't try to control the weather. It allows it. It witnesses it. It remains vast enough to hold it all.

Be the sky. This is mastery.

CHAPTER 5 – FIGHT FEAR

"There is no greater illusion than fear. Whoever can see through fear will always be safe."—
Lao Tzu, Tao Te Ching. 600BCE

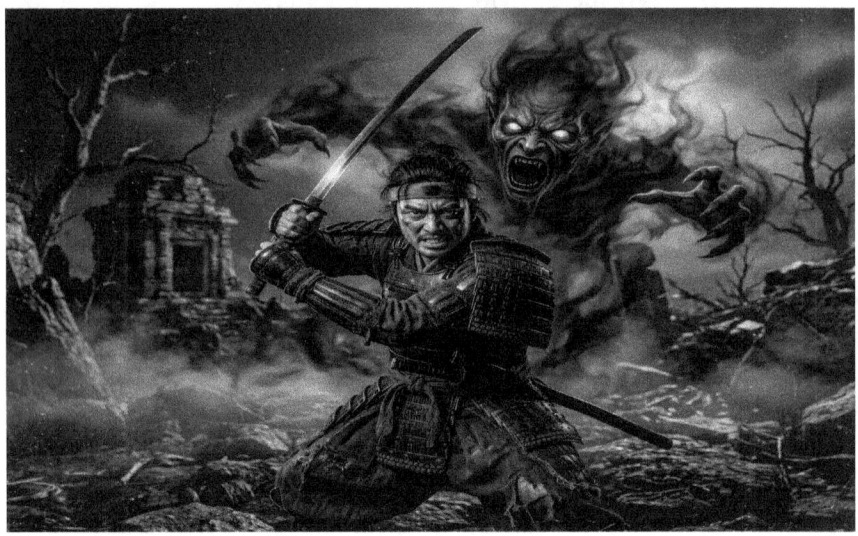

Fear is an Ally

If you get a bad feeling, trust your intuition, make your excuses, and leave. Your instincts are hardwired and they are meant to alert you to the unseen. Emotions are the most palpable connection to the spiritual realm that swirls around us. It does not serve us to bury information, instead we must process in an almost third party state, and this is the place from where we can decide and act without overthinking. The feeling of fear is a powerful early warning system. Fear is not debilitating if you can seize on it and take appropriate action in response to it.

I have always fought scared. I like it a lot now, but I didn't used to. When I was young, and without experience it was terrifying to be in a conflict of any sort. After some wins and some losses, the fear became less frantic and instead when it appeared, it jolted me to be at the highest level of attentiveness and alertness. I was still getting scared, but it transformed into a familiar emotional rush to get switched on. Later, the anticipatory fear, a whole body tingling became a pulse of excitement that I looked forward to. Eventually, I longed for the buzz of electric soul vibration of being fully present in the moment. Fear became a powerful drug, whose high was alluring and enticing that I went looking for.

Martial artists chose to face fears head on, and challenge themselves through constantly operating in progressively higher doses of it. Most untrained people spend their lives trying to avoid fear. They build gated communities, install double locks and alarms, metaphorically and in reality. They organize their entire existence around not feeling afraid. Martial arts training offers proven techniques to reduce and control fear by transforming it from a paralyzing force into actionable energy. Fear must be controlled—whether faced, reduced, eliminated, or redirected to serve as fuel. Through consistent martial arts practice, students learn to feed off the fear of conflict, channeling its energy and adrenaline rush into focused aggression and precise technique. This approach embodies the legendary Japanese samurai, Miyamoto Musashi's principle of "treading on the sword"—attacking decisively even as an opponent launches their opening moves, thereby surprising the aggressor and reversing their perceived advantage. Attacking first, quiets fear.

Fear has a Voice

I ask: What's more dangerous than fear itself? Answer; Ignoring it; burying it and letting it fester.

Gavin de Becker, one of the world's leading experts on violence prediction, describes this in his book, The Gift of Fear: "A woman is waiting for an elevator, and when the doors open she sees a man inside who causes her apprehension. Since she is not usually afraid, it may be the late hour, his size, the way he looks at her, the rate of attacks in the neighborhood, an article she read a year ago—it doesn't matter why."

What matters is what happens next. Does she trust that feeling? Or does she tell herself she's being paranoid, that she's overreacting, that she shouldn't judge people?

De Becker continues: "Every day, people engaged in the clever defiance of their own intuition become, in mid-thought, victims of violence and accidents. So when we wonder why we are victims so often, the answer is clear: It is because we are so good at it." De Becker uses this and similar examples to highlight how humans, unlike animals, often disregard their intuitive signals of potential danger due to a desire to be polite or logical, which can lead to perilous situations.

We are trained from childhood to be polite, to not make judgments, to give people the benefit of the doubt. These are good social skills. But they can get you killed when your intuition is screaming that something is wrong. Wild animals, conversely do not second guess their instincts, if they get a sense something is off, they act without hesitation.

Warriors understand this: fear is a tool, and it needs to be controlled, understood, and kept in its place—but never ignored.

The goal of martial arts training is to turn weakness into strength—not just strength, but mental and emotional strength. All three in harmony. Fear doesn't disappear through training. It transforms from paralyzing terror into excited anticipation. When you know deep inside that a fear has been addressed, it may come up during stressful situations, but your internal confidence will chime in and push the concern aside with a firm statement — we've trained hard on that and it won't be a problem. When I hear that voice in a time of need, I instantly feel encouraged.

Courage is trained. It is a mantra, a feeling that changes from terror to excitement and happy nervousness. Looking forward to the challenge, feeling prepared and anxious to get the action started.

Ultimate Fear

If we could totally remove the fear of death, there would be nothing scary in the natural world. But the reaper's constant shadow follows human existence. We're always marching toward our last days alive, slowly but surely approaching the final end of our mortal coil. That feeling can get terrifying if we have to face death close up.

In the limited time we have left—which is always getting shorter—and when death isn't immediately looming, the runner-up fear we all face daily is the fear of loss. Loss of time, reputation, respect, money, a pet, a friend, our health, etc. So we must deal with the constant risk of loss every day, but how? To fight the fear of loss means letting go of the idea that we have any control or ownership of anything past ourselves and our own emotions. To remember to enjoy and cherish, at every opportunity, the limited time we have with those very things that we are terrified to lose.

How do we control fear? Martial arts training develops self-awareness of physical movement, controlled breathing, and concentration, which helps overcome emotions produced by traumatic events—fear and anger—allowing practitioners to remain calm under stressful situations and respond appropriately. Here are the key exercises the martial arts employs to abate the fear response in practitioners;

Controlled Breathing Techniques Practice box breathing:

inhale for 4 counts, hold for 4, exhale for 4, hold for 4. Do this for 5–10 minutes daily. This activates your parasympathetic nervous system and trains your body to stay calm under pressure.

Progressive Exposure Identify something that makes you mildly anxious and deliberately expose yourself to it in small doses. Gradually increase the intensity over weeks. This builds tolerance and proves to your brain that feared outcomes rarely materialize.

Cold Exposure Take cold showers or end your regular shower with 30–60 seconds of cold water. The initial shock triggers a fear response, and learning to breathe through it trains mental resilience and physiological control.

Visualization Practice Spend 10 minutes imagining yourself successfully handling a feared situation. Engage all your senses—what do you see, hear, feel? Your brain can't fully distinguish between vivid imagination and reality, so this builds neural pathways for confident responses.

Physical Exercise Engage in vigorous exercise that elevates your heart rate. This familiarizes you with the physical sensations of stress (rapid heartbeat, heavy breathing) in a safe context, making them less alarming when they occur during actual fear.

Name and Label Emotions When fear arises, verbally identify it: "I'm feeling anxious about X." This simple act engages the prefrontal cortex and reduces amygdala activation, giving you more control.

Tests on martial artists unveiled that training produces profound effects on the amygdala, which processes emotions and fear responses. Karate training showed improved neural efficiency and stress tolerance. Martial arts practitioners exhibit better control over their autonomic nervous system—the fight-or-flight response—compared to non-practitioners.

F.E.A.R.

Fears manifest in different forms. Performance fear expresses as internal dialogue: "This is too hard. I can't do it." Physical capability fears can be acute, especially in front of others, where you could be humiliated in challenges of strength or coordination. So what is fear, and the fight or flight response? Fear is truly an emotional state, not rational or logical. But it has very real physiological manifestations that you must understand to control. Let's get into the science.

A stressful incident triggers the body's automatic activation of the sympathetic nervous system which can be both an asset and a challenge. When fear takes hold, the hypothalamus—the chemical command center of your brain—dumps a cascade of stress hormones like adrenaline and cortisol, that produce well-orchestrated physiological changes. The stress also makes your heart pound and breathing quicken. Muscles tense, beads of sweat appear, breathing accelerates, blood pressure and heartbeat change instantly. The dilation or constriction of key blood vessels can alter eyesight and muscle movements. While these adaptations evolved to enhance survival, they can interfere with the refined motor skills and tactical thinking required in martial arts—causing shaky hands, tunnel vision, auditory exclusion, and a deterioration of fine motor control.

The acronym F.E.A.R.—False Evidence Appearing Real—captures a fundamental truth about how our minds manufacture threats that don't exist. Much of what we fear never materializes, yet our brains treat imagined catastrophes with the same urgency as immediate danger, flooding our bodies with stress hormones over scenarios that exist only in our heads. We rehearse disaster, predict rejection, and catastrophize outcomes based on incomplete information, past wounds, or stories we've told ourselves so many times they feel like facts. The evidence appears real because our minds are extraordinarily convincing storytellers, painting vivid pictures of failure, humiliation, or loss that may feel inevitable. But appearing real and being real are vastly different. When you pause and examine your fears objectively—asking what you actually know versus what you're assuming, what's probable versus merely possible—most crumble under scrutiny. The job isn't to become fearless but to recognize when you're being manipulated by false evidence, to distinguish between legitimate warnings and mental fabrications. Real threats demand action. False evidence demands only that you stop believing it. A key to identify false fear is to watch for indecisiveness. Watch for incessant prioritizing of "what if" instead of dealing with "what is." The paralysis of analysis is fear disguised as prudence.

Small Exposures

Experienced martial artists train extensively to function effectively under this stress response, using techniques like controlled breathing, scenario-based sparring, and progressive exposure to high-pressure situations. This training helps practitioners maintain composure, execute techniques with precision, and make strategic decisions even when their nervous system is in overdrive. Rather than trying to eliminate the fight-or-flight response entirely, skilled fighters learn to channel its energy productively while minimizing its negative effects, transforming a primitive survival mechanism into a competitive advantage.

This understanding is the foundation on which martial arts training is designed at its core level: to help the practitioner take control of their body through practice, discipline, and focus. To win anything in the exterior world, first we must conquer the interior world.

Jeff Wise, author of Extreme Fear: The Science in Danger, explains that persistent exposure to anxiogenic stress—situations that trigger fight/flight—causes structural changes to the brain over time. These changes show up in scans and result in concrete cognitive modifications, specifically affecting how strongly people react emotionally to everyday events. So the constant small exposures to fear inducing stimuli are proven to reduce the overall emotional effects of the fear response.

Imagine a fear scale broken from mild concern to frozen terror. We all have this scale inside us, but through experience and internal wiring, each of us applies that range differently depending on perspective and experience.

Complete terror for a little girl might be seeing a spider versus an adult man thinking nothing of it. That same man might feel total terror being upside down in a tight culvert as water rises. Is either wrong in how they feel? It's relative.

We grow at different levels of capacity throughout our journey. Hopefully, as we age and gain experience, our scale widens and we leave childish fears behind as we face bigger and bolder challenges to our bravery.

Inoculation Training: Building Immunity to Fear

Clinical inoculation works by introducing small, controlled doses of a pathogen to build systemic immunity. The body learns to recognize the threat, develops defenses, and becomes progressively resistant. Fear responds to the same principle. Small, controlled exposures to what terrifies you create psychological antibodies. Each dose builds tolerance. Each survived encounter strengthens your resistance. Over time, what once paralyzed you becomes manageable, then routine, then conquered.

Small exposures leading to bigger encounters and with each step faced, progressively will compound confidence. But to be done properly, it needs a measured approach. It's systematic, slow and steady. It's progressive. It's scientific. The warrior who masters inoculation training doesn't eliminate fear—

they build such high tolerance that fear becomes background noise instead of a siren.

Active Progression

Start where you can barely handle it. Not where it's comfortable—that's too easy and builds nothing. Not where it's overwhelming—that's too hard and risks reinforcing the fear. Find the edge where your hands shake slightly, where your breath quickens, where every fiber wants to retreat but you can still force yourself forward. That's your starting dose. Let's think about some common fears and the application of the method.

Tight Spaces: From Closet to Culvert

If enclosed spaces trigger you, start with a closet. Door open, lights on, thirty seconds. Just sit there. Feel the walls closer than normal. Notice your breathing. Stay put. Next time, door cracked, twenty seconds more. Then door closed, light on. Then door closed, light off for brief intervals. Each session, one variable harder.

Graduate to crawling under a desk. Then through a cardboard box tunnel you built. Then into a car trunk—lid open at first, then briefly closed. Each time, extend the duration. Each time, remove one comfort element.

Move to actual confined training: low crawling under barriers, navigating tight corridors in full gear, squeezing through gaps that compress your chest. Now add complexity: do it wet. Do it in the dark. Do it with a task to complete while confined. Do it upside down.

The final test looks nothing like the first step. You're navigating a dark culvert, water rushing past, upside down in a harness, maneuvering through an obstacle course where the ceiling is inches from your face and the walls press against your shoulders. You're doing it because you've done variations of this a hundred times before, each one slightly harder than the last. The fear is still there—you just have immunity to its effects.

Heights: Rung by Rung

Acrophobia doesn't surrender to willpower alone. It surrenders to repetition and incremental elevation.

Start on a stepladder. Two rungs up, both hands gripping tight. Look down. Stay there until your pulse settles. Next time, three rungs. Four. Five. When the stepladder is routine, find a taller ladder. Six feet, eight feet, ten feet. Stay longer each time. Force yourself to look down, to shift your weight, to reach with one hand while the other holds.

Graduate to platforms. Low diving boards. Second-story windows. Fire escapes. Each time, stand at the edge longer. Look over more deliberately. Control your breathing while your body screams retreat.

Now functional height work: climb and descend fixed ropes. Rappel down structures of increasing height. Conduct tasks at elevation—not just standing there, but moving, working, solving problems while high off the ground. Cross narrow beams between platforms. Traverse hand-over-hand on horizontal ladders suspended in air.

The progression ends when you can fast-rope from a helicopter, conduct operations on tower cranes, or move across rooftops with the same mental state you have walking down a sidewalk. Not fearless—but immune to fear's paralysis.

Water: From Pool Laps to Chaos

If churning water and ocean mayhem trigger panic, you don't start in the surf. You start in the shallow end.

One lap, freestyle, controlled breathing. Then two laps. Five laps. Ten laps without stopping. When that's routine, swim underwater. Half the pool, then full length, then multiple lengths. Get comfortable with breath control and the sensation of your lungs burning while submerged.

Add stress: treading water for extended periods. Swimming in clothes, then boots, then full gear. Underwater breath-holding competitions with yourself—extending the time each session. Now simulate problems: swim while bound, navigate underwater obstacles, retrieve objects from the bottom.

Move to open water when the pool is routine. Lakes first, where the water is still. Then rivers with mild current. Practice swimming across current, not just with it. Get tumbled, learn to orient yourself when you don't know which way is up.

Graduate to surf: small waves first, just getting used to being pushed around. Then larger surf, where you practice duck-diving, getting through the break, recovering from being rolled. Get comfortable with chaos, with being unable to breathe when you want to, with being tossed and not knowing where the surface is.

The final iteration is full mission profiles in hostile water: night swims in cold ocean, with gear, through heavy surf, while exhausted from a full day's training. The terror that would have drowned you on day one is now just another environmental factor to manage.

Physical Contact: From Touch to Combat

If the fear of violence, of being hit, of physical confrontation makes you freeze, you must systematically desensitize yourself to contact and controlled aggression. This fear is primal—getting hurt violates every survival instinct. But warriors can't flinch when contact is inevitable.

Start with light contact drills. Partner up with someone you trust. Let them push you, not hard, just enough to move you. Feel the contact. Don't react defensively yet—just absorb the sensation of someone applying force to your body. Graduate to light slap boxing. Open hands, no power, just getting used to hands coming at your face. Blink less each session. Flinch less each round.

Now incorporate controlled sparring with protective gear.

Headgear, mouthguard, gloves. The first few sessions, you'll tense up, close your eyes, turn away. That's the fear talking. Keep showing up. Round after round, the sting of getting tagged becomes familiar. You learn that getting hit isn't the end of the world—it's just data. Adjust. Counter. Continue.

Increase intensity gradually: lighter gloves, harder contact, longer rounds. Remove one piece of protective gear at a time until you're working with minimal protection. Add scenario training: defend against multiple opponents, fight when exhausted, engage in positions of disadvantage. Get taken down. Get mounted. Learn to survive and escape from the worst positions.

The final progression is full-contact sparring and live scenario training where failure means you take real damage. You're not imagining violence anymore—you're in it. And because you've built immunity through hundreds of previous exposures, each progressively harder, you don't freeze. You don't panic. You execute.

The warrior who's been hit a thousand times in training doesn't fear the first punch in a real fight. They've been conditioned. They have antibodies against the paralysis that physical threat induces.

Social Confrontation: From Avoiding to Engaging

Many fear verbal confrontation more than physical. Start by simply holding eye contact longer than comfortable. Progress to speaking up in groups when you'd normally stay quiet. Practice saying "no" firmly to small requests. Graduate to controlled confrontations—returning bad service at restaurants, addressing someone cutting in line. Role-play aggressive verbal encounters. The final stage is handling actual hostile confrontations—de-escalating aggressive drunks, talking down threats, maintaining frame when someone is trying to intimidate you. The fear of social confrontation gets systematically dismantled.

Each of these follows the same protocol: minimum viable dose → repetition until routine → increment difficulty → repeat. The martial application is clear—warriors must function in conditions that would paralyze civilians. The only way to build that capacity is systematic exposure and progressive hardening.

The Inoculation Mindset

Every progression follows the pattern:

1. Identify the fear trigger
2. Find the minimum viable dose—the smallest exposure you can barely handle
3. Repeat that dose until it becomes routine
4. Increase one variable: intensity, duration, complexity, or discomfort
5. Repeat until that's routine
6. Scale again

Never skip steps. Never increase too fast. Not a sprint; it's a slow and systematic immunity building. Each exposure must be survivable, must be controlled, must add one degree of difficulty to what you've already mastered.

The warrior's advantage isn't natural fearlessness—it's manufactured tolerance. You've been in worse. You've done harder. You've survived scarier. Not because you're special, but because you've systematically inoculated yourself against the paralysis fear wants to inflict.

Document Your Doses

Keep a log. Write down each exposure, each increment, each survived encounter. This serves two purposes: it prevents you from plateauing too long at one level, and it provides proof of progression when your mind tries to convince you that you're not improving.

"Two weeks ago I couldn't keep my eyes open in a dark

closet for sixty seconds. Today I belly-crawled through a drainage pipe for twenty meters."

"Last month I flinched every time a jab came near my face. Today I took fifty clean head shots and stayed in the pocket."

That's immunity building in real-time. That's the inoculation protocol working.

The Endpoint

The progression never makes you immune to fear entirely—that would be psychopathy, not warriorship. What it does is raise your threshold so high that normal fears don't register, moderate fears become manageable, and even extreme fears can be processed and pushed through.

You still feel it. You just have enough antibodies built up that fear can't infect you with paralysis anymore.

One small dose at a time. One rung higher. One lap further. One step deeper into what scared you. One more punch absorbed and returned.

This is how you eat the elephant. This is how you beat paralysis. This is how you transform from someone controlled by fear into someone who controls fear.

Bite by bite. Dose by dose. Victory by small victory.

"Cowards die many times before their deaths; the valiant never taste of death but once."—William Shakespeare, 1599

CHAPTER 6 – EMBODY RESPECT

"A samurai should always respect his enemy. A samurai respects the enemy before and after the fight. If he kills an opponent, he is respectful to the corpse."—Inazo Nitobe, Bushido. 1899

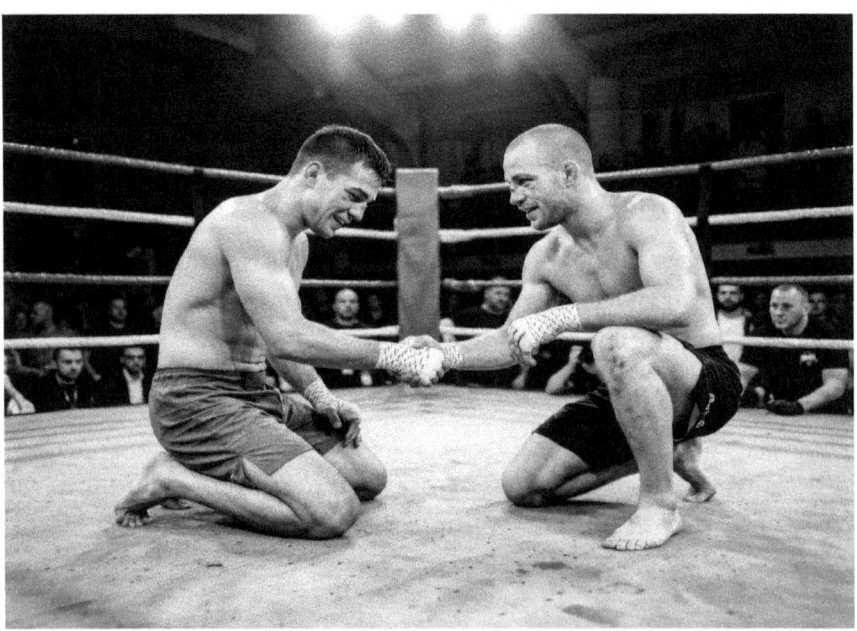

Warrior's Code

There is a code among warriors. In Japan, it has long been known as the eight principles of Bushido. In Bushido are enshrined the ethics of the samurai warriors based on morals and virtues, such as courage, loyalty, and honesty. The fourth principle is Rei—Respect.

It is easy for a seasoned warrior to respect the hard work and discipline of another warrior. It is the recognition of the difficult journey that all warriors must walk. But respect in Bushido goes deeper than mutual recognition between fighters.

It is all–encompassing respect. Respect for those who take the time to train with you and help you grow. Respect for the long hours and sacrifice in life choices required to walk the path. Fitness of body, mind, and spirit is a difficult balance to uphold consistently, week over week, year over year.

I often train privately with other instructors. Coach Darren MacDonald is one of my favorite trainers. I learned many valuable lessons over the years. In one session, I was in guard and from mounted, he knee cut, then incredibly fast for a big man of 6'2, 260lbs, flat chest spun 180° until his thighs were clamped around my face. He then wiggled his legs until his thighs were slapping my cheeks. I was stunned and he took the moment of confusion to slip me into a knee bar. It was fast and effective. It was unexpected, and slightly offensive! I had never heard, seen or experienced anything like it before, and it was an excellent lesson. Sure, we respect each other before and after the match. But during the contest, it is about winning and dominating, using unconventional weapons of mass disruption (in this case his thighs), and having fun with exploring new twists and combinations to techniques.

Darren is a quintessential warrior, an intuitive ring and street fighter, an instructor with incredible patience and a strict training regime that has never wavered in the 25 years I have known him. A hard worker who has produced tangible and admirable results.

The more established and known the warrior is, the more respect they command. But this respect isn't demanded—it's earned through consistent action over time.

Your Word Is Your Bond

When I was very young, my father told me to always keep my word. No matter what.

Being an honorable, trustworthy person will separate you from all others. If you want respect, earn it. You do not want people to fear you—you want their respect, support, and love. Fear is taxing and fleeting. Love and respect only grow over time. Want to have an army behind you? For every person you keep your word to, your army builds by one.

Data confirms this principle extends far beyond martial arts into every area of success. Surveys about business leadership consistently show that integrity—defined as keeping commitments and following through on promises—is the supreme quality for leadership. Companies with high levels of trust outperform their competitors by nearly three times in total returns to shareholders.

When you keep your word, you make "trust deposits" in an account with every person you deal with. People see you as reliable and honest. Over time, this compounds. If others can rely on you to come through no matter what, you will be ushered into the inner circle of influential and powerful people as your reputation for honor grows.

The data is stark: 58% of employees trust a stranger more than their own boss. This reveals a massive trust deficit in our world. So many people break their word casually, make promises they don't keep, and wonder why opportunities don't come their way.

Warriors understand differently. Your reputation is more valuable than money. Your integrity is worth more than your career. When you practice making the right decisions consistently, eventually it becomes a habit. Then it becomes who you are.

"The supreme quality for leadership is unquestionably – integrity. Without it, no real success is possible, no matter whether it is on a section gang, a football field, in an army, or in an office." — Dwight D. Eisenhower. 1962

Foundations of Self-Respect

Respect your family line. The blood that flows through you was earned and fought for. In your lineage, your forefathers gave up many things, fought many battles, sacrificed so that your blood could continue. No family is perfect, but your bloodline survived despite often difficult odds—and that in itself is a testament to those warriors who came before you.

Respecting your ancestors and their history is respecting yourself, and you should respect yourself in all ways.

Personal Respect

"A man who honors his parents and his teacher, honors himself."—Grandmaster Byung Kyu Lee, 2005

To have respect for others, you must first possess respect for yourself. If you do not love yourself, you cannot truly love others, and the same goes for self-respect. When others see you respect yourself, they will follow that lead. No one can know how to treat you properly if you don't set the standard that is expected.

Building self-respect starts with how you treat your own body and time. Maintain your physical health—eat nourishing food, get adequate sleep, and move your body. Not out of punishment or vanity, but because you deserve to feel good and function well. Honor your boundaries and say no to commitments that drain you or compromise your values. Respect your time and don't get distracted from your goal. Watch out for time burglars! Recognize that protecting your time and energy isn't selfish—it's essential. Don't apologize for having limits. Your body and your hours are the only resources you truly own, so guard them accordingly.

Equally important is how you relate to the people around you. Remove toxic influences and distance yourself from people who consistently diminish, manipulate, or disrespect you. Your presence in someone's life is a privilege, not a right. Respect your privacy—keep your inner self secure from gossip and information leaks. This will translate to not dealing in gossip about others. Following the Golden Rule is paramount for respect. The company you keep shapes who you become, so choose relationships that elevate you rather than drain you.

Finally, cultivate the internal dialogue and habits that build genuine self-worth. Keep promises to yourself and follow through on commitments you make to yourself just as you would for others. If you say you'll exercise, or write, or rest, do it. Your word to yourself should mean something. Speak to yourself with kindness—notice your internal dialogue. Would you talk to a friend the way you talk to yourself? Replace harsh self-criticism with the same compassion and understanding you'd offer someone you care about. Invest in your growth by dedicating time to learning, developing skills, or pursuing interests that matter to you. This shows you believe you're worth the investment. Celebrate your wins and acknowledge your accomplishments, even small ones. You don't need external validation to recognize your own progress and effort.

Sadly, there are those that think admitting mistakes damages self-respect. The opposite is true. Admit when you're wrong. Owning mistakes shows self-respect because it means you value integrity over ego. It takes strength to be accountable to yourself. Despite best efforts, you may not always make the right decisions, but self-respect demands that you go back and fix mistakes where possible and make them right.

Hard Work Fosters Self-Respect

Martial arts training reveals something profound about self-respect: it's built, not inherited. Practitioners show significant increases in self-esteem following training interventions. But here's what matters—the improvement comes from doing hard things consistently, not from affirmations, praise, or positive thinking. Self-respect, like all forms of respect, is earned.

You can't think your way into self-respect—and that's why hollow self-esteem exercises fail. You earn it by keeping promises to yourself. By showing up when you don't feel like it. By doing the work when no one is watching.

After studying Tae Kwon Do for eight weeks, female participants reported higher self-esteem compared to control groups. In one study, clinically depressed subjects were enrolled in a six-month judo program, and the new students reported increased self-worth following the intervention. The mechanism is clear: martial arts training develops self-regulation through meditation, self-evaluation, and rewards for practice and self-discipline. The lesson? Hard work increases the amount we value ourselves.

Work at skills that are hard and cannot be faked. You will know the value of your efforts, and those who have examined closely what you are accomplishing will also know the effort required. Their respect of you will climb.

Learn your body and how to use it. Work at martial skills that take obvious rigorous study. Make it a great reason to learn a flashy move worthy of the movie screen. Not for the practicality, but for the sheer pleasure of performing it with style. Building your self-worth and being proud of your efforts and accomplishments is a process and a journey.

The best judge of your efforts is your own honest, conscious, critical review.

Align the Public and Private Self

Integrity takes its truest form here. The word comes from Latin—integritas, meaning wholeness, soundness, completeness. When your actions align with your values, when your private self matches your public self, you have integrity. When they don't match, you feel the dissonance. That feeling is your internal warning system telling you you're off course.

Consider the executive who preaches work-life balance in company meetings but answers emails at 2 AM and expects the same from subordinates. Or the social media fitness influencer posting inspirational training content while skipping workouts for weeks at a time. These people present one face to the world while living another reality in private. The split creates internal tension—a constant, exhausting performance that drains energy and erodes self-respect. They know the truth about themselves, and that knowledge creates shame, anxiety, and the perpetual fear of being exposed as frauds. Notice how the lack of character manifests: not as dramatic moral failings, but as the quiet corrosion *of living a lie.*

Now consider the martial artist who trains when no one is watching, who practices the same respect in their living room that they show on the mat, who treats strangers with the same courtesy they show their instructor. Their public and private selves are unified. There's no performance, no mask to maintain, no fear of exposure because there's nothing hidden. What you see is what exists.

When these two selves merge—when your public face reflects your private reality—you achieve alignment with the Tao, the natural flow of existence. Embracing honesty in its purest form: not just telling the truth to others, but living truthfully with yourself. The internal conflict disappears. The exhaustion of pretending vanishes. You experience wholeness because you are actually whole, not fragmented across competing identities. This unity brings profound well-being—the deep peace of knowing that who you are and who you claim to be are the same person. No dissonance. No shame. No fear. Just integrity, lived completely.

Company You Keep

Don't be with people or do things that will make you feel regret, or risk you losing respect for yourself.

The problem with being around people who do not respect themselves is they will continuously put you in circumstances that risk your own self-respect—and they will do it to you on purpose. They don't want someone around that makes them feel bad or forces them to face their own failures and lack of self-esteem.

The people around you should be those you hold in high regard—people who evidence having and producing admirable actions and results. You are fundamentally shaped by the six people you spend the most time with. We become who we socialize with, elevate, and emulate.

The Lakes study (2004) on martial arts practitioners establish this principle clearly. The training environment matters as much as the training itself. Martial arts schools that emphasize respect, formal etiquette, and cultural values tied to their styles produce practitioners with improved self-esteem and determination. The community reinforces the values.

Further, the seminal Lakes (2004) research examining martial arts as sports-based mental health interventions found that the emphasis on complex, repetitive movements, self-controlled behavior, and interpersonal respect were common factors in programs that successfully reduced externalizing behaviors and built psychological benefits.

You can't build honor in a dishonorable environment. You can't develop self-respect surrounded by people who mock discipline and reward laziness. The warrior chooses their companions carefully, knowing that who you spend time with shapes who you become.

If your circle doesn't challenge you to be better, find a new circle.

Paradoxes of Judgment

As long as you try to impress others, you reveal you're not convinced of your own strength. As long as you strive to be better than others, you question your own worth. As long as you try to elevate yourself by lowering others, you doubt your own greatness. These are the paradoxes that trap most people in a lifetime of insecurity masked as ambition and this will not produce respect for others or yourself.

The person at peace with themselves doesn't need to prove anything. They know their worth without requiring validation. They recognize their own greatness and let others keep theirs—understanding that someone else's brilliance doesn't diminish their own light. This is the inner confidence you seek.

Most people never reach this level. They spend entire lives comparing, competing for status, trying to prove they matter by diminishing someone else. They measure their diamond against others instead of polishing their own. They're so busy looking sideways they never look inward, and is the antithesis of the warrior path.

The martial arts teach something radically different: your competition is yourself yesterday. Your enemy is your own weakness, your own hesitation, your own compromises with excellence. The scholar within you studies your patterns. The warrior within you disciplines your actions. The lover within you cultivates compassion for your own imperfections while refusing to accept them as permanent. When these three operate in balance, external comparison becomes irrelevant, and your self-respect will grow.

Ancient warriors knew intuitively: engagement in combat training positively influences well-being through sequential processes. Physical activity generates positive emotions, which contribute to stress relief, which builds ego-resilience over time. But—and this is critical—the effects depend on the quality of your participation, not just showing up. The more genuine your engagement in training, the greater the effect on self-esteem. This suggests that internal focus, not comparison with others, drives the psychological benefits. You're not there to be better than the person next to you. You're there to master yourself.

When you stop seeking external validation and start building internal standards, everything changes. The anxiety drops away. The need to posture disappears. You can give genuine respect to others because their excellence doesn't threaten yours. Their success doesn't diminish your potential; it proves what's possible.

Recognize what true confidence looks like. Not arrogance. Not bravado. Not the fragile ego that shatters when challenged. Quiet certainty. Real self-respect.

Perfection Is Not the Goal

When practicing, do so with all your heart and energy. Train so that your efforts win respect from yourself and all those in audience. Be impressive to you and them. All done through effort, not flair.

Try to understand the reason for a technique and customize it for your body. Execute techniques with precision and style. In this way you mark your life and the way you performed in it as a person who respects their time and is committed to excellence.

But perfection is not the goal. Doing your best and improving is.

Perfection costs time and is an exercise in diminishing returns. The longer you spend in one area, every other area must pay the price. Try as hard as you can, continue to work on all areas, and accept the results. Move on and accept good enough as long as you put in all you have for the best results. Perhaps an area of contention and I recognize the potential disconnect. Let balance in all things be your guide here. Meditate on it for personal clarification.

One must be adult enough to know when to let challengers and challenges go. Goals are not written in stone that all must be completed or it is a failure. Everything has its place and time, and some new goals or challenges may need your full attention and take precedence over your current plans.

Life is short. To make the most of your experience, there needs to be a realistic view of priorities and circumstances. Life is full of sacrifices, and unclear future outcomes make being decisive in the fog of war and limited information difficult. Some goals need to be surmounted with more pressing challenges.

Research found that martial arts training promotes characteristics associated with well being including greater autonomy, emotional stability, assertiveness, and self-assurance. But the training also teaches acceptance—acceptance of where you are, acceptance of the long road ahead, acceptance that mastery is a lifetime pursuit, not a destination.

Completing stages of martial training and having official recognition is not unlike graduation from university, or being promoted, given a rank or other honors. They can be transformative moments. But nothing can replace when you earn your own respect. When deep inside you know what you did was hard and you are proud of yourself for sticking to it and achieving a goal. It reminds you that sacrifice and perseverance will give results.

A Belt Is Just Cloth

Rank isn't everything, and being less advanced than others

is a good place to face new challenges and challengers. It is okay to be the underdog, there is no time like the present to test yourself. The one with the most to prove often becomes a celebrated champion because there was so much to overcome that the experience gives everyone hope. Through hard work, dedication, and being the most improved student, you can achieve goals and dreams faster than if you politely, "waited your turn.". A lesson across all genres and applications. Rank alone should never hold you back from attempting greatness and reaching for the stars.

The belt around your waist is just cloth. The rank is just recognition. What matters is what you know you did to get it. The private victories—the mornings you showed up exhausted, the techniques you drilled until your body moved without thinking, the moments you wanted to quit but didn't.

Those are what build self-respect. Not the external symbols.

This principle extends to every area of life. The degree on the wall doesn't make you educated—the learning does. The job title doesn't make you a leader—your actions do. The wedding ring doesn't make you a good spouse—your daily choices do.

External validation is nice. But it's hollow without the internal foundation. Build the foundation first. The external recognition will follow, and when it does, you'll know you earned it.

Anger is Poison

"Holding on to anger is like poisoning yourself and hoping someone else will die." — Buddha. 598BCE

Self-respect is destroyed by anger. When you carry resentment, grudges, and old wounds, you're choosing to disrespect yourself in the most fundamental way—you're allowing past events and other people's actions to control your present state.

You're giving them power over you long after the moment has passed. Every minute you spend replaying old slights is a minute stolen from building your future. Why keep memories that work against your success?

Anger is often triggered by the pain of past experiences. Identify the cause of your anger and its triggers to reduce involuntary reactions in times when intelligent decisions are required. The same applies to resentment and grudges. They eat you from the inside. They cloud your judgment. They make you predictable to your enemies and exhausting to your friends. It is the opposite of respect—both for yourself and for those around you who must deal with your volatility.

Respect yourself enough to release what doesn't serve you. Every ounce of energy you spend on old anger is energy you can't use for present challenges. When you hold grudges, you're declaring that your past is more important than your present, that your wounds define you more than your potential. That's profound self-disrespect disguised as righteousness.

The Martial Arts Difference

Following the tenets of martial arts develops self-control and enhanced awareness of personal boundaries, which creates measurable psychological benefits. training alone reduces the hormones associated with anger and aggression—true across all athletic disciplines. But martial arts goes further. The combination of disciplined training, meditative practice, and the intentional cultivation of respect produces benefits that extend far beyond what conventional sports offer. You're not just conditioning your body; you're training your nervous system to choose measured response over reactive emotion. You're literally rewiring yourself to select respect over rage.

Here's where martial arts diverges sharply from every other competitive sport: competing black belts consistently maintain lower levels of verbal hostility and assaultive behavior compared to practitioners of equally intense physical sports that lack a historical doctrine. Football players, hockey athletes, boxers without martial warrior guidelines—they channel aggression into performance, but that aggression often spills beyond the arena. Their training has no self-control mechanisms. Martial artists, by contrast, are replete with the culture of respect that permeates from their essence.

Why? The answer lies in what's taught from day one, from the moment you tie on a white belt. Martial arts doesn't just teach you how to hurt someone—it teaches you why not to. The respect drilled into every bow, every kata, every sparring session isn't ceremonial window dressing. It's the core curriculum. You learn respect for yourself: that your integrated self are instruments requiring care and discipline. You learn respect for your craft: that the techniques you're mastering carry real consequences and demand serious responsibility. You learn respect for your opponent: that the person across from you has endured the same grueling path, faced the same fears, earned the same hard-won skill.

This understanding is profound and personal. When you've felt the pain of a perfectly executed technique, when you've tapped out, when you've been humbled on the mat—you carry a visceral knowledge of what you're capable of inflicting. And paradoxically, this knowledge breeds restraint. You respect your opponent because you understand intimately what it took for both of you to be here. The years of training. The injuries. The mental battles. The moments of wanting to quit. This mutual recognition creates a bond that doesn't exist in other sports, where opponents are obstacles to overcome rather than fellow travelers on the same difficult path.

This dynamic isn't mirrored *anywhere* else. Not in conventional athletics. Not in team sports. Not in individual competitions without a martial foundation. **Only in the martial arts.** Why? Because only martial arts deliberately integrates the capacity for violence with the philosophy of peace. You're taught to be dangerous *and* disciplined simultaneously. The art makes you capable of harm while the philosophy demands you avoid it. This tension—this paradox—is what separates martial artists from every other type of competitor.

Choosing advanced self-respect: knowing that you are capable of violence but asserting control. Knowing that you could dominate but choosing to show restraint. Having devastating power but exercising it only when absolutely necessary. Anyone can rage—it requires no skill, no discipline, no character. Anger is easy. Violence is simple. But it takes a true warrior to remain calm when provoked, to possess lethal capability and keep it sheathed. Calmness in the face of provocation is the ultimate demonstration of self-respect because it proves you control yourself, not your emotions. And when you demonstrate that level of mastery, you command respect from others—not through intimidation or aggression, but through undeniable presence, capability, and restraint.

The person who respects themselves doesn't need anger as a weapon. They've developed something far more powerful: control.

More Respect, Less Conflict

Respect yourself, and others, and you improve your fighting record by reducing the fights that are only about social strife. Then you can focus on the fights that matter.

Most conflicts are avoidable. Most violence is preceded by multiple opportunities to de-escalate. Most arguments are fueled by ego, not genuine threat.

When you have genuine self-respect, you don't need to prove anything in pointless confrontations. You can walk away without feeling diminished. You can let insults slide without feeling disrespected. You can choose your battles because you're not constantly fighting to defend a fragile sense of self.

The better you get at fighting, the less you need to fight. Your confidence is genuine, not compensatory. Your presence communicates capability without words.

Exhibiting the ultimate form of respect: respecting yourself enough not to waste your time on meaningless conflicts, and respecting others enough to give them the benefit of the doubt until they prove they don't deserve it.

The warrior trains for war but seeks peace. The training isn't contradictory to the goal—it's the foundation of it. You can only choose peace from a position of strength. Weakness that avoids conflict isn't peace, it's fear.

True respect—for yourself and others—comes from knowing you could fight but choosing not to. Not because you're afraid, but because it's beneath you.

Respectful equals Successful

Success is the culmination of respect working in harmony across three dimensions, each one inseparable from the others.

Self-respect is the foundation. Without it, nothing else holds. You can't build external success on internal chaos. This means setting goals and keeping promises to yourself with the same rigor you'd apply to a contract with someone you deeply respect. The private victories come first: showing up, doing the work, maintaining standards when no one is watching. Your internal integrity—the alignment between who you claim to be and who you actually are in private—determines everything that follows.

Respect for others means keeping your word and building trust through consistent action. Your reputation is your most valuable asset in any arena. When people know they can count on you absolutely, doors open that remain closed to others. Trust is the currency of all human interaction, and you build it one kept promise at a time. Here's the deeper truth: keeping your word to others is simultaneously an act of self-respect.

When you honor commitments to others, you're proving to yourself that your word has weight, that you are who you say you are. The public and private self align. Integrity in action.

As you develop real capability, as you produce real results, as you demonstrate real integrity—respect compounds naturally. Success breeds success. The reputation you build through consistent action creates opportunities that accelerate further success. But this only works when it's genuine, when it's earned through actual achievement, not performance or posturing.

Experience across business, military, and academic institutions confirms this model. Honor codes effectively promote integrity and reduce unethical behavior—but only when people have genuine commitment to them, not just lip service. That commitment comes from seeing the code lived, not just written. From being part of a community that values honor through action, not just words. In business, leaders who embody integrity inspire the same in their teams, creating a ripple effect that elevates entire organizations. But this only works when the integrity is real—when actions match words consistently over time, when the leader respects both staff and organization enough to practice what they preach.

The warrior path teaches this through direct, unforgiving experience. You can't fake your way through a sparring match. You can't pretend you put in the training hours. You can't talk your way out of a real fight. The mat doesn't lie. The opponent doesn't care about your excuses. Results reveal truth. Martial training builds not just physical capability but psychological resilience and self-efficacy—you're proving to yourself through concrete action that you can overcome real challenges, that your commitments to yourself and others mean something tangible.

Only real work produces real respect. Only hard-earned capability commands genuine trust. Only authentic integrity

—the complete alignment of your three selves: scholar, lover, and warrior—creates the foundation for lasting success.

This brutal honesty—this direct feedback loop between effort and results—is what makes martial arts such an effective teacher of respect and integrity. You learn that shortcuts don't exist. That your word to yourself matters most. That genuine capability commands genuine respect.

Ring Fight

I was in the corner coaching a talented young fighter in a Vancouver tournament. Just before the match began, he had the look in his eyes that told me he needed some encouragement. His opponent was a beast and this was going to be a tough match. Confidently, I told him he was going to win, and I was sure of it. He was all ears. I asked him if he believed in God. He said yes, so I told him the guy in the other corner doesn't believe in God. Therefore, it will be two against one, because God will be in the ring with you, and that guy will be in there by himself. My fighter processed, and I watched in his eyes as his energy settled into calm determination. It was a tough fight, but he won.

Only One Fear Allowed

It has been said the only fear worth keeping is the fear of God. Pascal's wager, if you will.

Pascal's argument goes like this: If you believe in God and God exists, you gain everything (eternal salvation). If you believe in God and God doesn't exist, you lose little. If you don't believe in God and God exists, you lose everything (eternal damnation). If you don't believe in God and God doesn't exist, you gain little. So fear of God is the best of the balance of risk vs. probabilities with the greatest outcomes in your favor. Therefore, I resubmit, the only fear worth keeping is the fear of the highest power.

If God is the only fear you have, then respect for the divine provides the moral foundation for everything else. All human respect—for yourself, for your family line, for your teachers, for your opponents—flows from recognizing something greater than yourself.

It's not about religion versus secularism. It's about understanding that respect requires acknowledging value beyond your own immediate desires. Whether you call it God, the Tao, universal energy, natural law, or human dignity—there must be some principles you hold sacred that constrains your actions even when no one is watching.

Without this, "respect" becomes mere calculation. You keep your word only when it benefits you. You treat others well only when they can hurt you. You maintain standards only when someone is checking.

That's not respect. That's transaction.

When no one is Watching

True respect—the kind that builds lasting success, deep relationships, and internal peace—comes from knowing that how you act matters independent of consequences. That there is a right way and a wrong way. That your character is defined by what you do when no one will ever know.

The warrior code exists because warriors understood this principle thousands of years before modern psychology proved it. Honor isn't optional for success—it's foundational. Self-respect isn't self-indulgence—it's self-mastery. Respect for others isn't weakness—it's strength.

Respect transforms through training from an abstract virtue into lived reality. From something you're told to do into something you choose to be. From external expectation into internal standard.

Every time you keep your word when it costs you something, you prove to yourself that your integrity isn't for sale.

Every time you treat someone with respect who can't benefit you, you show that your values aren't transactional. Every time you hold yourself to a high standard when you could cut corners, you build the foundation of genuine self-respect.

This accumulates. Small choices become habits. Habits become character. Character becomes destiny.

The difference between a warrior and everyone else isn't superior genetics or lucky circumstances. It's the daily choice to embody respect—for yourself, for others, for the path itself.

They rise to the standard they set for themselves, even when no one is watching.

Especially when no one is watching.

CHAPTER 7 – HONE THE PHYSICAL

"Pain is the best teacher, but no one wants to take his class."—Choi Hong Hi, 1978

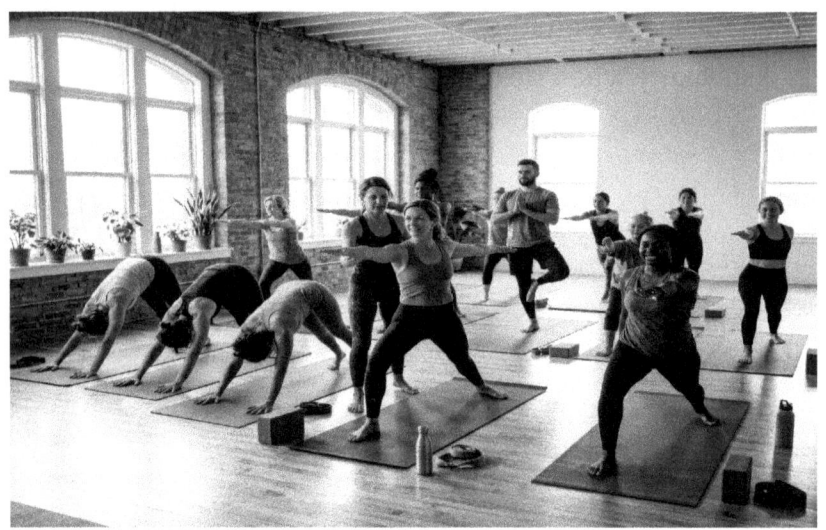

Great warriors exude their inner strength. Effort equals results. The chiseled physique of the warrior and the predator like movements are forged in the fighter's mind and manifest in the physical realm. Take a moment to imagine seeing yourself in the mirror, ripped and shredded with low body fat and defined, rippled muscles glistening in the light. If you visualize it, you can make it happen.

Your Body Is Your Only Permanent Possession

You will be given a body when you are born. You may like it or hate it, but it is the only thing you are sure to keep until you die, so you had better learn to take care of it.

There are no shortcuts and there is no replacement for sheer effort. Put in the time and reap the rewards.

If you zoom out and look at your body as a single functioning organism, and you sculpt and train and nourish each part of it from head to toe, you will function as a cohesive unit and heal and build as a collective.

Your body is the same as a business, or a family, or a society. Each part needs to operate at its peak capability to not be the weak link that fails the whole.

We have the choice to accentuate the gifts we are born with and work to improve or compensate for the weaknesses. There is no telling how high you can go with your gifts polished and your weaknesses known, admitted, itemized, and targeted for improvement.

Learn your body and how to use it. Learn to dance, how to skateboard, try new things and don't hold back. Your physicality improves as you explore all the ways to move your body and all the unique skills you can learn to do with it. Bend, twist, and explore.

Train Your Body to Tolerate Pain

Pain is information. Your body telling you something needs attention. But in combat, pain is also a weapon your opponent uses to break your will.

Warriors train their bodies to withstand pain that would stop ordinary people cold.

It is not about being tough. It's about biology.

Probes on exercise-induced hypoalgesia—the reduction in pain sensitivity following exercise—reveals that both aerobic and resistance training actually change how your nervous system processes pain. A single bout of dynamic circuit resistance exercise produces increases in pain tolerance of 15–20% at exercising body areas. Regular training amplifies this effect over time.

The mechanism is fascinating. When you exercise intensely and repeatedly, your body adapts. Training induced hypoalgesic adaptations, marked changes in the central nervous system and immune system. In other words, your pain threshold literally rises through consistent exposure to controlled stress.

Martial artists have known this for centuries. Makiwara boards for hardening knuckles. Rope conditioning for shins. Sand training for hands. Modern science confirms what traditional training methods discovered through trial and error: repeated exposure to controlled pain desensitizes the nervous system's response.

Conditioned pain modulation works on a simple principle: pain inhibits pain. By training through moderate discomfort regularly, you raise your baseline tolerance. When the fight comes, what feels excruciating to your opponent registers as manageable to you.

It isn't about becoming numb. It's about expanding your capacity to function under duress.

Athletes achieve heightened pain thresholds and tolerance compared to normally active individuals. But this advantage isn't hereditary—it's trained. Performers in combat sports show significantly higher pain tolerance because they've logged thousands of hours pushing through discomfort during training.

The tactical advantage is clear: if you can fight effectively while hurt, and your opponent cannot, you win. The moment they're focused on their pain is the moment they're not focused on defense.

The critical point fact-finding reveals: you must train smart. Exercise that produces acute hypoalgesia is often perceived as moderately painful—around 5 or 6 on a 0–10 scale. Push past that into injury territory and you compromise future training. The goal is consistent exposure to manageable stress, not random acts of self-destruction.

Breath Is the Foundation

"You control your spirit with your breathing."—Hirokazu Kanazawa. 1989

If your breathing is slower, your clarity is higher. Working on great cardio and reducing the chance of lactic acid buildup increases clarity during times of stress. A calm heart equals a calm mind, and a calm mind makes better decisions faster.

Controlled breathing in combat sports isn't just automatic —it's prudent. If you find yourself in an overwhelming situation and start to hyperventilate, mentally queue in on your breathing. Control your breath and you will think more clearly. Slow down your breathing and focus on this first, it is the priority. The comprehensive deteriorate fast if you aren't getting oxygen from deeper, slower breath.

I was swimming from a boat to a rocky wave break in the ocean. The sun was hot and the small waves of salty water were warm and all was right in the world. I didn't have fins, only a cheap mask with a built in snorkel. All of the sudden as I got within 10 feet of the rocks, an undercurrent held me in place, the harder I swam the less I moved. The waves rocked me in place and I was running out of breath and energy. I tore the mask off and gulped air, this started the hyperventilation cycle, and I started to sink under each wave. Time slowed and the pause happened. I knew I first needed to get my breathing under control or I wouldn't be able to muster my last strength and get to shore. I quickly went inside my mind and prioritized slow breaths and timing forward motion with the waves. The breath slowed, the gulping and choking stopped and with my last ounces of strength I swam, kicked and clawed my way onto the rocks. I got pretty cut up and bruised on the rocks but was grateful for the resting spot. It was a close call, and it happened quick. Takeaway – wear a damn life jacket, even if you don't think you need it.

BreathWork is Training

When your mind and body move as one unit, when breath synchronizes with movement, when intention flows directly into action without hesitation—this is cultivating Qi (or Chi). A state where technique becomes effortless, where complex sequences execute without conscious thought, where you respond to threats before you consciously perceive them. Cultivating Qi by deep concentrated breathing begins the cycle for power enhanced combat focus. This ancient mind–body exercise is practiced by the monks of Shaolin temple, whose feats of incredible endurance and strength are legendary. These concepts sound esoteric, but they describe something concrete: the integration of mental intention with physical execution. If this interests you, I encourage the reader to explore this subject in greater detail with a Qi-gong master for further exposure to the techniques.

At its core, breathing is about oxygen—the critical element muscles need during intense physical exertion. Oxygen plays a pivotal role in aerobic metabolism, the process that generates energy required to sustain prolonged activity. In combat sports where endurance is key, maximizing oxygen intake is vital.

But equally important is the expulsion of carbon dioxide. High levels of CO_2 in the blood cause a drop in pH, leading to muscle fatigue and impaired cognitive function—a fighter's worst enemies. Effective breathing techniques help regulate

CO2 levels, maintaining the delicate balance needed for peak performance.

Diaphragmatic breathing stands as the fundamental technique, often distinguishing great fighters from good ones. Your diaphragm is the most efficient muscle in your body for breathing. The abdominal muscles help move the belly up and down, giving you more power to fill and empty your lungs completely.

Military trials on combat athletes show that inspiratory muscle training—resistance breathing exercises—produces significant improvements in pulmonary function. Six weeks of resistive breathing training increased maximum voluntary ventilation by 28.6% in MMA athletes. That's measurable improvement in your engine's capacity.

For more proof review the incredible journey of Bas Ruuten. Bas trained himself from an asthmatic and sickly kid to one of the greatest ring fighters from the K1 series using innovative ideas like breathing through mouth-guards with small holes cut in them while doing heavy cardio and running hills.

The connection between breathing and performance psychology is equally profound. Psychologists confirm that different emotions generate different forms of breathing. When you're calm and focused, your breathing is regular, deep, and slow. When you're anxious or angry, your breath becomes short, fast, irregular, and shallow.

Here's the powerful part. When you control your breathing patterns, you can **shift your body into different emotional states**. Slow, controlled breathing sends a signal to your brain that you're not in danger. You'll start to feel physically calmer almost immediately. Heart rate decreases, blood pressure drops, and clarity sharpens. So breathing with purpose can change your emotional state!

Breath control must be the first thing to master under stress.

Breathe smoothly to stay calm—in through your nose, out through your mouth. Maintain consistent breathing rhythm, especially under pressure. Shallow chest breathing leads to rapid fatigue. Deep diaphragmatic breathing sustains you through the longest rounds.

Combat athletes who incorporate breath work into their routine present much better ability to control heart rate and muscle recovery over time. Regular practice allows you to sit down and almost immediately put your body into a state of controlled readiness. The longer you practice, the more efficient your breathing becomes and the better your body adjusts to stressful situations.

Breath control keeps your heart-rate in check and while you are under pressure, this means keeping it in the performance zone. The secret to mastering breathing is practice. Don't wait until fight day to implement breath work. Train it like any other skill, because under pressure, you will default to what you've practiced.

BPM Matters

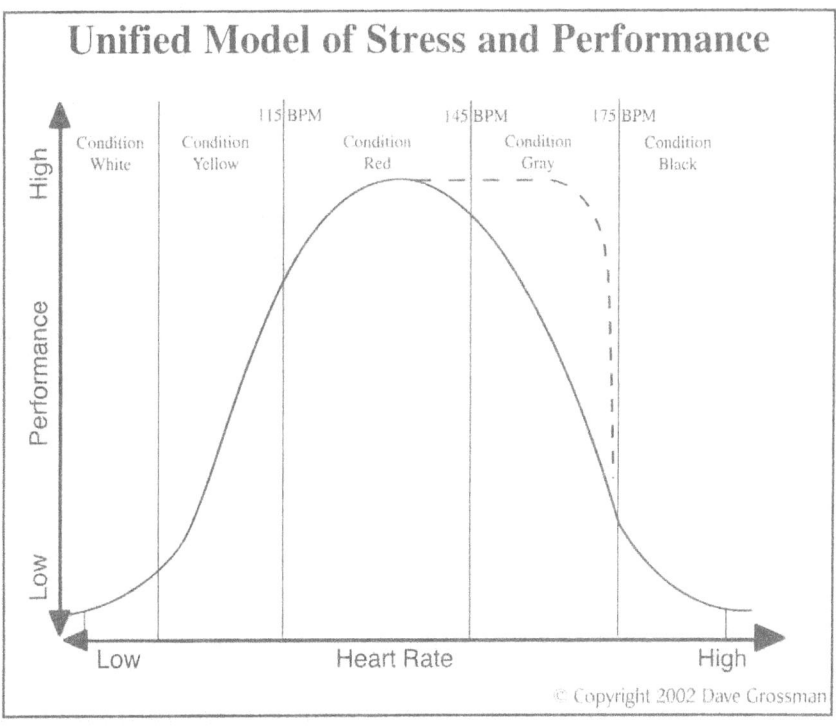

Lt. Col. David Grossman's Unified Model of Stress and Performance gives us a scientific method for understanding what we've always known instinctively in the dojo: training under pressure makes the difference between freezing and fighting back. The diagram shows a clear relationship between your heart rate, your physiological state, and your ability to perform under stress. At rest, you're in Condition White—relaxed but not very effective. As your heart rate climbs into the 115–145 BPM range (Condition Yellow and Red), you enter the performance zone where your body and mind work at their peak. But push past 175 BPM into Condition Gray and Black, and everything falls apart. Your fine motor skills disappear, tunnel vision sets in, and complex decision-making becomes nearly impossible.

We have found where martial arts training earns its keep. When chaos erupts—whether it's a real threat or just the pressure of sparring in front of your peers—your body wants to spike straight into Condition Gray. Your heart hammers, your breathing goes shallow and rapid, and suddenly the techniques you've drilled a thousand times feel like they're locked behind a door you can't open. But consistent training does something remarkable: it teaches your nervous system that elevated stress isn't a catastrophe. Through progressive exposure to controlled pressure, you learn to stay in Condition Red even when adrenaline floods your system. The breathing exercises we practice aren't just warmup rituals—they're tactical tools that let you regulate your heart rate and keep yourself in the performance zone when it matters most.

The beauty of this model is that it explains why we train the way we do. Kata and shadow boxing build the foundation when your heart rate is low. Drilling with a partner adds moderate stress. Live sparring and scenario training push you closer to real-world intensity. Each level teaches your body to maintain technique and tactical thinking at higher heart rates. When someone who's never trained faces violence, their system redlines immediately into Condition Black. But you? You've been there before. You've felt your heart pounding at 150 BPM and still executed that combination. You've learned to breathe through the chaos. That's the targeted physiological conditioning as revealed by Grossman's research. Your training keeps you in the zone where you can actually perform when everyone else is physiologically incapable of doing anything but panic. At least, that's our plan.

To Failure and Beyond

Train to maximum rep, to failure, beyond when your mind wants to give up—it wants to preserve some fuel in the tank. Hit reserve and go to total exhaustion. Leave it all on the dance floor.

You will be more confident knowing you did the most in training—more than anyone else would.

This principle seems brutal, but it's essential. you will tell you to quit long before your body actually fails. The gap between "I can't" and true physical incapacity is vast. Warriors close that gap in training so they know exactly how much they can endure under pressure.

When you've trained to true failure repeatedly, you know with certainty that when the fight gets hard, you have more left. You've been to that place before. It's not unknown territory. It's familiar ground where you've proven you can function.

This doesn't mean training recklessly. It means occasionally—not every session, but strategically—pushing past the comfortable stopping point to discover what you're actually capable of. These are the sessions that build unshakable confidence.

Fighting is Training

The best way to be prepared for the fight is, surprise, fighting. Your body doesn't truly understand what it needs until pressure tests it. Sparring reveals weaknesses no mirror can show you. Hard rounds expose cardiovascular gaps your roadwork missed. Getting hit teaches tension management no meditation alone can provide. The fight itself is the forge—it doesn't just test the body, it hones it.

It is said that only the dead have seen the end of war. In times of peace, the warrior wisely prepares for war. The fight lasts minutes. The preparation takes years. When the time to perform arrives, the time to prepare has passed. But understand this: every sparring session, every hard round, every time you step into live conflict is preparation *and* refinement happening simultaneously. Your body adapts to what you demand of it. Demand fighting, and it becomes a fighting body.

Violence doesn't ask permission. It doesn't wait for you to be ready. The fight picks you—in a parking lot, at a gas station, outside a bar when you're walking away. You don't start it. But you will finish it.

Reading the Pre-Fight

An enemy leads with intention before they lead with fists. You'll feel it first—the shift in energy, the predatory focus, the closing of distance. Trust that feeling. It's older than language.

Watch the legs. They telegraph movement before hands reveal intention. The body shifts weight before it throws a punch. The shoulders drop before the tackle. Read these signals and you're already two moves ahead.

In that moment between recognition and action, know this: they chose this. You're simply responding. The moral high ground is yours. The spiritual advantage is yours. The legal justification is yours. They initiated. You're defending. Never forget that distinction.

The Decision Point

Must you wait for the first blow? No. When threat becomes imminent—when closing distance meets hostile intent—preemptive defense is righteous defense. The law recognizes this. Your survival demands it.

Strike first if you must. Strike hard. Strike with complete commitment. There's no such thing as a half-measure in violence. If you've decided to engage, then engage fully. Hesitation gets you hurt.

But understand: response, not aggression. Defense, not attack. You didn't seek this fight. The fight sought you. That clarity matters—legally, morally, spiritually.

Execution Principles

Be mentally prepared for a long struggle even if you hope for a short one. Fights are exhausting. Adrenaline lies about how much you have left. Pace yourself even in chaos. Breathe, slowly, calmly, deeply, even in the storm. Here's where your conditioning shows itself—not in how hard you can go for ten seconds, but whether you're still functional at minute three when your arms feel like concrete and your opponent is still coming.

Stay loose until the split second your strikes make contact. Tension before impact wastes energy and telegraphs intention. Relaxation conceals. Explosion at the point of contact—that's where power lives. This looseness under pressure? You can't fake it. You can't drill it in shadow boxing alone. It comes from being hit, from returning fire, from learning your body's response to real threat.

Strike in combinations. Let one action lead fluidly to the next until the threat stops. Flow from strike to control. Adapt to what presents itself. Break them with speed and impact. Break their will to continue. Force them to quit mentally and collapse physically.

Keep it simple. One move after another as opportunities appear. Just do. Don't overthink. Don't hesitate. See the opening and take it. Your training will surface when your mind gets quiet.

Never move when you don't have to. If you must move, move the minimum necessary. Economy of motion preserves energy. Wasted movement invites counters. Efficiency is survival.

Mental Organization

Great fighters are great artists. They learn a style and make it their own, gracefully flowing and conforming to the opponent's movements. The mind commands and the body adapts —shifting, adjusting, accessing all resources at once and then one at a time. This adaptability is physical as much as mental. Your nervous system learns efficiency through combat, not theory. Your muscles learn when to fire and when to rest through the chaos of real exchanges. Fighting teaches yourself lessons the heavy bag never could.

In any confrontation, know the other person is scared. They're covering it with aggression, but fear drives them. Capitalize on it. They think you're scared too. Let them think it. Then show them otherwise.

It is best to seldom respond with violence. When you do, it's justified. It's necessary. You're not the aggressor. You're the one who tried to walk away. You're the one who didn't want this. But now that it's here, you'll handle it with the skill you've built and the calm you've cultivated. Be of great cheer, you are about to build and cultivate more!

A warrior has grit, toughness, conditioning. A warrior is not pampered, entitled, emotionally fragile, or cowardly. A warrior stands ground when ground must be held.

Concern yourself only with the ultimate goal: neutralizing the threat and getting home safe. Everything else is distraction. Your ego doesn't matter. Looking tough doesn't matter. Winning the argument doesn't matter. Survival matters. Safety matters. Going home to your people matters.

The best defense is not needing it. The second-best defense is ending the threat quickly and decisively when defense becomes necessary.

When violence finds you, respond like the warrior you've trained to be—and remember that every time you respond, every time you test yourself under pressure, you're not just using your training. You're refining it. The body you bring to the fight becomes sharper through the fight itself.

Core Strength: The Source of Explosive Power

Plyometric core training—explosive power is built from the twisting action . Each limb has a finite amount of potential kinetic energy, but coupled with the ability to throw your weight into every blow, the energy coefficient is multiplied several times over.

Core training should be the essence of your workout focus. You must strive to find new ways to engage the upper and lower abs and back muscles in harmony. With a strong core, speed plus mass equals power.

To have knockdown capability in one punch, you need to generate enough force to overwhelm the opponent's senses and stun their whole body into submission. You achieve this through cross-training and focus training.

While weight training builds sheer strength to overcome an adversary—to be able to pick them up and throw them down. Plyometrics focuses on "jump training," using exercises where you train muscles to exert maximum force in short intervals of time, with the goal of increasing explosive power (speed x strength).

Plyometrics conditioning enhances fast-twitch fibers as well as strengthening sinew and ligament response, which is the basis of muscle speed. Isometric holds, build the static strength to maintain torso position under pressure. Each part must be made strong so that whole is strong. Like a bundle of sticks, the stronger each stick is the stronger the bundle will be when they are all placed together as one. A complete warrior must also train so all the parts work well together and that means isolating down to train each part individually.

Think about the bio-mechanics of striking. The power doesn't come from your arm alone. It originates in your legs, transfers through your core rotation, and accelerates through your shoulder and arm to the target. Every link in that chain must be trained.

A weak core is a broken chain. All the arm strength in the world won't produce knockout power if your midsection can't transfer force from your legs to your upper body efficiently. Maximum power is generated from employing as much as possible from any given position.

Train the twist. Train trunk rotation. Train for stability under resistance. Train your core from every angle until it's an unbreakable axis around which your entire body pivots. I bet the "Twist" dance of the 1960's would be good cross-training for this.

Meditation Is Training

Meditation– Sit quietly. Focus on breath. When thoughts arise (they will), notice them and return to breath. You're not trying to stop thinking. You're training your attention to remain where you place it instead of being dragged by every mental distraction.

This directly translates to fighting. The ability to stay focused on your opponent instead of the crowd, the judges, your fear, your ego. Ten minutes of daily meditation builds that muscle.

Mokuso (Pre-Training Meditation)– Before training, sit in seiza or cross-legged for 1-2 minutes. Eyes closed. Breathe deeply. Leave the day's stress outside. Enter training with clear focus. This ritual creates separation—you're not bringing work problems or relationship drama, leave them behind.

Breath Control Under Pressure– When sparring gets intense, your breath gets shallow and rapid. Deliberately slow it down. Deep inhale through nose. Hold, 10 count. Controlled exhale through mouth–duration 10 count. This signals your nervous system: we're in control, not panicking. Oxygen flows. Heart rate drops. Decisions improve.

Post-Action Awareness– After sparring or competition, sit quietly for a few minutes. Don't immediately jump into analysis or conversation. Just sit with what happened. Feel it. Process it. This cultivates zanshin—the awareness that continues after the action ends.

Meditate as much as you stretch. Meditate and breath while stretching. Find the small spaces in your day to allow the universe to talk to you. Meditate when you can—during massage, while in the shower, while sipping coffee or tea, steal the quiet moments between activities to be still and listen.

Regular exercise combats anxiety by making humans less responsive to the stress hormone cortisol. Meditation amplifies this effect. Combined with training, meditation creates a comprehensive approach to managing the fear and stress responses that can sabotage performance.

Imagery and Visualization

Picture in your mind's eye performing a technique—a complex combination, a difficult transition, a perfect execution.

Imagine your body doing it over and over. As you visualize, your mind fires the associated synapses in your brain and activates the very muscles that would engage to perform the movement. Before training, mentally rehearse the exercises you know you'll do. See yourself moving through each rep, each drill, each sparring sequence. Then step onto the mat and make it physical.

Master Young was the first to teach me this principle. He explained that even while sleeping and dreaming, we can be training. "The mind doesn't stop practicing," he told me. "My grandfather taught my father this. My father taught me. Now I teach you." This wisdom had been passed down through generations of martial artists in his family, refined through centuries of practice—yet only recently confirmed by Western science.

Studies now validate what these masters always knew. Mental rehearsal, mental visualization, mental practice—whatever you call it—helps athletes reduce anxiety and improve performance by activating neural pathways and priming muscles for action. A 2004 landmark Cleveland Clinic study in the scientific journal "Neuropsychologia", found that training alone, without any physical exercise, increased finger abduction strength by 35% and elbow flexion strength by 13.5% over 12 weeks of practice—just 15 minutes per day, 5 days per week. The researchers concluded that training enhances the cortical output signal, which drives muscles to a higher activation level and increases strength. Through visualization alone, you can make yourself stronger!

When you visualize yourself executing a technique with granular detail—feeling the weight shift through your stance, hearing the snap of impact, seeing your opponent's body react—your nervous system fires neural pathways nearly identical to actual physical practice. This strengthens the mind–muscle connection and builds mental blueprints for complex movements before you ever throw the technique.

Master Song Young's grandfather didn't need a laboratory to know this worked. His masters had shown him. He tested it through decades on the mat. He passed it to his son, who passed it to his son, who passed it to me. The science simply confirms what generations of warriors already understood: the mind trains the body, even in stillness.

Stretching is Training

For body mastery you must be equally strong in every aspect. I refer to the Taoist mantra of training; using the left side and right side equally, creating body balance. Everything is a left–right, up–down flow. To punch with the hands effectively one must change levels constantly—punch high, punch low, the legs are doing as much or more than the arms. So in combat for one part of you to function at its peak, all other parts must also be ready trained, strong and flexible ready for the action.

But balance also means knowing when to rest and rebuild.

Yes, train hard—but rest hard. Do not over train. Stretch twice as much as you train. Stretch before, after, and on off days. Training data shows that proper recovery is when adaptation occurs. You break down muscle in training. You build it back stronger during rest. Avoiding fatigue and injury is just as valuable as training hard. Stretching helps you stay limber and keep muscles and ligaments at their most supple.

Lions sleep all day, get up only to stretch, and don't spend time jogging and hitting the weights to keep their fitness. They just stretch and yet are always ready to explode into action when needed. There's wisdom in that.

Stretching improves flexibility, reduces injury risk, enhances blood flow, and promotes faster recovery. Dedicate serious time to mobility work. The fighter who can move in full range of motion has tactical advantages, specifically speed and resilience, that the stiff fighter can never access.

The Extra Mile

In the end, the best training for achieving excellence in martial arts is, surprise again, practicing the martial arts. If you train and spar every day, you will be better prepared for life's eventualities, if for no other reason than by being de-stressed from the consistent physical outlet.

But "taking care of the physical" involves all aspects—from nutrition to meditation, to self-care like skin brushing, hanging, working out, and embracing life with hope and a positive attitude. Anything you can do to assist your journey in the positive should be considered and implemented. One extra sit up, one more meditation. Ten minutes earlier to bed. It all counts for points, your health points.

Think of creative ways to make an exercise harder and more challenging. Look at all the types of predicaments you might find yourself in and train from those places. Give yourself experience in every possible problem and look for methods to get better at finding solutions quickly. Push yourself a little more all the time and find opportunities in problems.

Experimentation consistently shows that varied training produces more adaptable athletes. When you train only one way, you become skilled in narrow circumstances. When you train in multiple positions, multiple scenarios, multiple energy systems, you develop the adaptive capacity to handle anything.

Your body is the vehicle through which you experience life and accomplish your goals. Treat it with the respect it deserves. Challenge it regularly. Feed it properly. Rest it adequately. Push it past perceived limits occasionally to discover its true capacity.

More Sweat in Training, Less Blood in War

The more effort you put in when there is little on the line, the better you will do when everything is at stake. Ego, honor, or life itself. Why not keep your odds high that no matter the circumstance you can keep all three? Going one more round, staying late to work on a technique, finding new training partners who have notable accolades and fighters with skills you desire. Doing the minimum won't get you far, only doing the extras will. When you train, train with purpose. Train with intensity. Train as if your life depends on it, because someday it might.

Athletes who train with high perceived effort and intentionality show greater improvements than those who just go through the motions at the same workload. The mental component of training matters as much as the physical stress. Bring your authentic best to your workout. When you step on the mat, leave the world behind. Be present. Focus completely on the work at hand. Make every rep count. Make every round matter. This focused practice is what separates warriors from people who merely work out.

This integration is trained through thousands of hours of deliberate practice. Through breathing exercises that connect state to physical performance. Through meditation that quiets the mind's interference with the body's instincts. Through sparring that forces real-time decision-making faster than conscious thought allows.

The goal is automaticity—where technique bypasses conscious processing and springs directly from trained reflex. Where your body executes perfectly because you've programmed it through relentless repetition.

The highest level of training arrives where the comprehensive become indistinguishable, where training has wired your nervous system to respond optimally without requiring thought.

The physical preparation you've done—the pain tolerance you've built, the breathing patterns you've mastered, the core strength you've developed, the thousands of reps you've logged—this creates rational confidence. Not arrogance. Not bravado. Calm certainty that you've done the work.

When you know you've trained harder than your opponent likely has, when you know you've been to the edge of your capacity and survived repeatedly, when you know you will function under stress because you've tested it there—this knowledge produces unshakeable confidence tempered by healthy respect for the challenge ahead.

The warrior mindset: prepared but not rigid, confident but not careless, ready to adapt to whatever the fight demands because your physical preparation has been comprehensive enough to handle the unexpected.

"In times of peace, the warrior wisely prepares for war." We train diligently in the hope that we need to risk our lives the fewest times possible. But if necessary, we have the best chance of winning when called upon.

The body is the vehicle. The mind is the driver. Breath is the fuel. Training is the road map.

Hone them all. Leave no weak link. Build a physical foundation so solid that when the storm comes, you stand unshaken.

CHAPTER 8 – FUEL THE VESSEL

"With health, man has a thousand hopes, without it he has but one."—Confucius. 488 BC

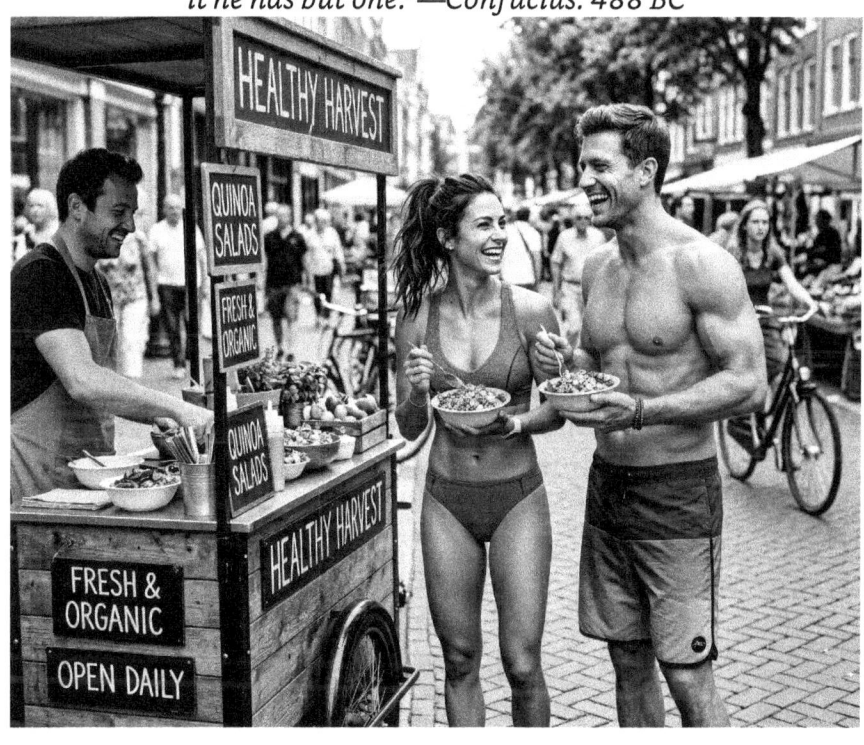

You Are What You Eat

Confucius told us that with health, man has a thousand hopes. But health doesn't come from wishful thinking, it comes from what you put in your body. There are many excellent books on nutrition, and what follows is a warrior's overview of the essentials. I encourage you to seek out information as specific to your body type/blood type as possible. But remember this universal truth: you are what you eat.

Health is not found in the doctors office nor in a prescription pill jar. Quacks have been putting mercury and lead as fillings in teeth, spraying babies with DEET, giving pregnant mothers thalidomide, and using leeches to bleed sicknesses out. Sure, these are old news stories, but in their day they were considered the pinnacle of cosmopolitan health care. I remember clearly the advertising when I was young, "4 out of 5 doctors smoke camels.", and sugary, hyper processed cereals were "fortified with vitamins" for a nutritious start of the day. From seed oils to aspartame, there are endless examples of once promoted additives that are suddenly banned when long term effects are proven to be harmful. There is no reason to assume what you are being told/fed today is any better. History may not repeat, but it definitely rhymes.

The bottom line is you are responsible for every single thing that goes into your body, regardless of who told you it was good. If you choose to put garbage foods in, you can expect poor performance. Garbage in, garbage out. I recommend raw whole foods that are as close to their original form and meddled with by man the least. If you see an ingredient list of more than five words you do not recognize, best to find a more direct form of nutrition.

Think of it this way: your body and your integrated self

are built and run like a car and its engine. Your performance is the result of the fuel you burn. If you had a Lamborghini, Ferrari, or Jaguar and you needed fuel, would you choose the best top-rated highest quality or the cheapest gas available?

The comparison should be obvious. In today's world of processed food, food dyes, and chemical coloring, many of us are putting the cheapest fuel in our bodies, causing all kinds of poor performance problems—both short-term and long-term, cumulatively.

The easy list of foods to avoid: anything with sugar, processed fats, oils, or chemicals. Stick to raw, unprocessed, and unadulterated non–genetically modified food sources.

With the Western world's slick marketing, addictive formulas, and cheap products with long shelf lives it can be difficult. I've tried to keep my intake to a balanced diet of organic and raw foods to the extent that I built and operated a small hobby farm to supply my food for many years.

In proteins, I like to have salmon, chicken, and steak at least once each a week. I picture the salmon as giving me agility, the chicken speed, and beef bringing strength. If I want to focus on one of those qualities, I'll double up that week. I am a huge sushi fan so a majority of my fish is eaten raw. Studies have shown a reduction in nutritional value when foods are cooked and heated. Consider minimizing eating cooked food where practical and safe. Personal responsibility for your health means always making the best choices for today's goals and for your future self. There is something critical that many people do not know about eating times and nutrition. When you eat matters almost as much as what you eat, and there is an opportune time that nutrition is uptaken in the most advantageous and efficient way. Where the highest value and best return of your chew time is realized. When the castle door is wide open, vitamins, minerals, and all the unnamed phytonutrients will be put to highest and best use. The research is clear. The International Society of Sports Nutrition studied thousands of athletes and found a pattern: those who hit 20–40 grams of quality protein every three to four hours—like clockwork—built more muscle, dropped more fat, and performed better than athletes eating the same total amounts randomly throughout the day. Think of nutrient timing not as some narrow thirty-minute "anabolic window" but as a door of opportunity. That door stays open wider and longer than the old myths suggested. But here's what matters: if you train hard, if you train multiple times per day, if you have a life outside the gym—that peri-exercise period becomes your chance to actually hit your daily numbers. Miss that window and you're scrambling all day trying to catch up on calories and macros. It becomes impossible. The question isn't "before, during, or after?" The answer is "before, during, and after." All of it.

Here's What Works

Pre-exercise fueling for sessions lasting longer than 90 minutes: Load 1–4 grams per kilogram of bodyweight of carbohydrates in the hours before. Solid or liquid—bars, gels, energy drinks, fruit juice. Whatever your gut tolerates and your experience has proven. Test it in training. Never experiment on game day.

During exercise exceeding 60–90 minutes: Consume 30–60 grams of simple carbs in a carb-electrolyte solution every 10–15 minutes throughout the bout. It's not optional, it is a must. Blood glucose drops. Fatigue sets in. You're robbing yourself of performance. Sip consistently. Maintain the standard.

Post-exercise within 30 minutes to 2 hours: Approximately 1 gram per kilogram of carbs plus 0.5 grams per kilogram of protein. Quality food timed correctly is when recovery accelerates, when tissue repair happens and when adaptation begins. The castle door is wide open and the drawbridge is down—drive through it.

Protein consistently throughout the day: Every 3–5 hours. The old thirty-minute protein window myth? False. Muscle protein synthesis rates stay elevated for up to twenty-four hours post-training. But that doesn't mean you can slack off. Consistent protein intake—every few hours—maximizes your body's ability to build and repair. Feed the machine regularly or watch it sputter.

THE WARRIOR'S DAILY FEEDING SCHEDULE

The castle door opens widest when the sun is high. Plan your feeding windows to align with your body's natural rhythms and training demands.

TIME	PROTEIN	CARBS	PURPOSE	STATUS
6:00 AM	30-35g	1.0-1.5g/kg	Front-load calories	■ OPEN
9:00 AM	25-30g	0.5g/kg	Maintain synthesis	■ OPEN
12:00 PM	30-35g	1.0g/kg	Peak metabolic window	■ WIDE OPEN
2:00 PM	20-25g	1-4g/kg	Pre-workout fuel	■ OPEN
4:00 PM	0g	0.5-1.0g/kg/hr	Training fuel	■ OPEN
5:30 PM	25-30g	1.0g/kg	Recovery window	■ OPEN
8:00 PM	25-30g	0.5g/kg	Final protein dose	■ CLOSING
11:00 PM	0g	0g	Fast begins	■ CLOSED

DAILY TARGET FOR 70KG WARRIOR: 150-200g protein | 3-6g/kg carbs based on training volume

The Sun Knows What's Up

Tell me if you've heard this one; Breakfast is the most important meal of the day. Guess what? TRUE! In clinical trials, approximately 2.5 times more weight was lost when the majority of calories were consumed at breakfast rather than evening meals. Not 10% more. Not 25% more. Two and a half times more weight loss. Load up your food in the morning, and you have all day to burn it off.

THE BREAKFAST ADVANTAGE

Front-load your calories. The data proves it. Warriors who eat like kings at breakfast and paupers at dinner dominate those who flip the script.

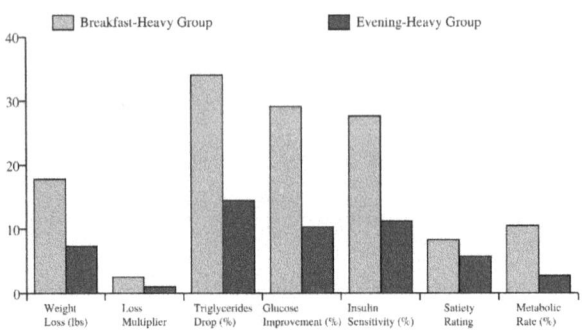

THE VERDICT: 2.5× more weight loss. 34% triglyceride reduction. Superior glucose control. The castle door opens widest at dawn.

The same study showed triglyceride levels decreased by 34%. Greater improvements in glucose control. Better insulin response, higher energy levels overall. Increased feelings of fullness and satisfaction, means less temptations for junk food mid-day.

Your body isn't designed to process a massive steak dinner at 10 PM while Netflix glows in the dark. It's designed to eat when the sun is up. When light hits your retinas, metabolic rate increases. Digestive enzymes flow. Insulin sensitivity peaks. Your circadian biology is wired for daytime feeding.

Fasting

Front-load your calories. Eat your biggest meals in the morning and midday. Let dinner be lighter, earlier. Then fast through the night while you sleep and recover. If you can stop eating by 6 pm and not eat again till 10 am the next day you will trigger autophagy. The minimum fast for effect is typically 16 hours, though some sources suggest it can start between 12 to 24 hours and becomes more significant after 24 hours. While shorter fasts may initiate the process, longer fasts, like 24 hours, can lead to a more significant cellular response. I mix daily fasts (16 hrs), with quarterly 36 hour fasts, and I do a major fast (72 hrs) once a year. You need to work out what is best for you and your body.

YOUR BODY'S METABOLIC CLOCK

Your metabolic rate follows the sun—not your schedule, not your convenience. Peak efficiency occurs when light hits your eyes. Fight your biology and you fight yourself.

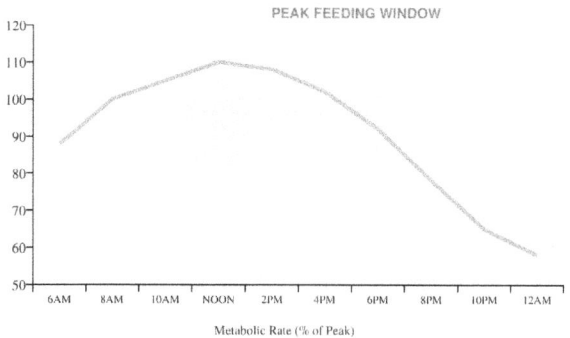

CASTLE DOOR STATUS:
- 6AM-4PM: Wide Open (88-110% efficiency)
- 4PM-8PM: Closing (78-92% efficiency)
- 8PM-6AM: Locked (58-78% efficiency)

THE WARRIOR'S DECREE:

Walk through the castle door when it swings widest. Feed your body in rhythm with the sun. Front-load your calories at dawn. Fuel your training with precision. Close the door at dusk and let recovery begin.

The castle door of opportunity does not wait. Neither should you.

This aligns with ancient wisdom about intermittent fasting and eating in rhythm with daylight hours. The ancients didn't have peer-reviewed journals and metabolic ward studies. They just observed that warriors who ate with the sun moved better, fought harder, recovered faster.

Science finally caught up with what the body already knew.

Train Hard. Eat Right. Time It Well.

The timing of energy intake and the ratio of macronutrients enhance recovery, augment muscle protein synthesis, repair damaged tissue, and improve mood states following high-volume or intense training. Not theory, but documented, replicated, peer-reviewed fact.

When you eat matters. Treat your nutrition with the same precision you bring to your training. Plan your feeding windows. Hit your protein targets. Front-load your day. Fuel your sessions properly.

The castle door of opportunity is open. Walk through it with intention.

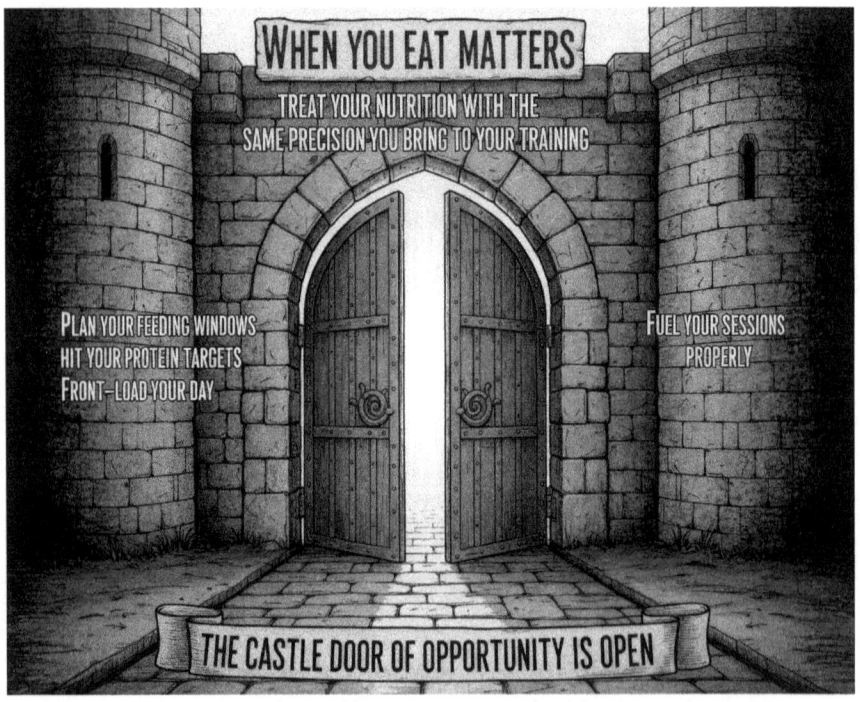

Technical Notes for the Serious Student:

For a 70kg (154 lb) athlete:

– Daily protein target: 140–175g (20–25g per feeding, 6–7 times daily)

- Training day carbs: 3–6g per kg bodyweight depending on volume (210–420g)
- Pre-workout: 70–280g carbs 1–2 hours before
- During: 30–60g carbs per hour for sessions over 60–90 minutes
- Post-workout: 70g carbs + 35g protein within 30min–2hrs
- Breakfast should contain 30–40% of daily calories
- Final meal should be completed 2–3 hours before sleep (finish at 6 pm, in bed by 9 pm)

Adjust these numbers based on bodyweight, training volume, and individual response. Test. Measure. Adapt. The warrior's body tells the truth if you're willing to listen.

Gut Microbiome: Your Hidden Performance Advantage

Your intestines and associated organs form a complex, interconnected system. Digestion affects your entirety—insides and out, all your energy, immunity, recovery, clarity. There is an entire ecosystem that supports your athletic performance and very existence, and it is the trillions of microorganisms living in your gut.

Elite athletes have different gut bacteria than average people. Their microbiomes are more diverse, more efficient at harvesting energy, better at managing inflammation, and stronger at maintaining the intestinal barrier that keeps toxins out of the bloodstream. No coincidence—it's cause and effect.

Certain beneficial bacteria convert exercise-induced lactate into fuel that powers performance. In clinical studies, mice inoculated with one of these strains (Veillonella) improved endurance by 13% and recovered faster from intense exercise. Athletes who train regularly develop richer populations of beneficial species like Bifidobacterium, Lactobacillus, Prevotella, and Faecalibacterium—bacteria that directly support muscle function, reduce inflammation, and improve nutrient absorption.

Your gut microbiome determines how much you gain from training. It influences muscle glycogen storage, antioxidant activity, lactate metabolism, and gastrointestinal integrity. It even predicts how much strength and cardiovascular capacity you'll build from the same training program compared to someone else.

Here's the practical part: you don't need expensive supplements if you're eating properly. Whole, raw, unprocessed foods naturally support a healthy microbiome; industrial processed foods, added sugar, pasteurization, microwaving, artificial additives, chronic stress, and unnecessary antibiotics destroy them. Fermented foods have a significant and positive impact on the gut microbiome and health in general, including increased short-chain fatty acid production and decreased bloating. Think about adding traditional fermented foods: kimchi, sauerkraut, kefir, yogurt with live cultures to your diet.

Quality food removes the need to intervene. Your body knows how to maintain its own ecosystem when you give it the right materials. Eat like your performance depends on it—because it does.

Your gut is not just your digestive system. It's a performance-enhancing system that requires deliberate cultivation.

Hidden Enemies: Parasites, Mold, and Infections

Most people walk around with compromised gut health and don't even know it. Parasites, mold exposure, and chronic bacterial infections silently sabotage performance, drain energy, and create systemic inflammation that prevents recovery.

Parasites are more common than you think. They're not just a third-world problem. Poor food handling, undercooked meat, contaminated water, and even your pets can introduce parasitic infections. Symptoms often masquerade as other issues: chronic fatigue, brain fog, digestive problems, unexplained weight loss or gain, grinding teeth at night, constant hunger despite eating.

If you've traveled internationally, eaten sushi regularly, consumed undercooked pork or beef, or have pets that go outdoors, consider getting tested. A comprehensive stool analysis can identify most common parasites. Treatment typically involves antiparasitic medications or herbal protocols, but must be done under supervision because die-off reactions can be severe.

Mold exposure is an epidemic in modern buildings. Water damage, poor ventilation, and sealed buildings create perfect environments for toxic mold. Black mold, Stachybotrys, and other species produce mycotoxins that damage mitochondria—your cellular energy factories.

Symptoms include: chronic sinus issues, respiratory problems, brain fog, fatigue that doesn't respond to rest, joint pain, sensitivity to smells, and mood swings. If you're training hard but feel worse instead of better, mold exposure may be the culprit.

Check your living and training environments. Look for water stains, musty smells, or visible mold. Test if necessary. Remediation must be done properly—trying to clean toxic mold yourself often makes exposure worse by dispersing spores.

Bacterial infections, particularly gut dysbiosis and conditions like SIBO (Small Intestinal Bacterial Overgrowth), wreak havoc on nutrient absorption and create chronic inflammation. You can eat perfectly and supplement religiously, but if your gut can't absorb nutrients, you're starving at the cellular level.

Signs include: bloating after meals, alternating constipation and diarrhea, food sensitivities that seem to multiply, skin issues like eczema or acne, and autoimmune symptoms. Breath testing can diagnose SIBO. Treatment involves specific antibiotic or herbal protocols followed by careful reintroduction of probiotics and healing foods.

Nutrition science shows connections between gut infections and mental health. Reports have found that schizophrenia and other psychiatric conditions can be triggered or worsened by chronic infections, parasites, and toxin exposure. The gut–brain axis is real. What happens in your digestive system directly affects your brain chemistry, mood, decision-making, and clarity.

For the warrior, clarity is essential. You cannot afford brain fog or compromised decision-making. Address gut infections aggressively. Your performance depends on it.

Electrolytes: The Body's Electrical System

Heart health and the cardiovascular system are of particular interest to athletes seeking peak physical performance. Blood pressure, the elasticity of veins, oxygenation of blood, and the strength of the heart muscle are of acute importance to performance but also to life itself.

The balance of potassium, magnesium, and sodium contribute to what are known as electrolytes—minerals that perform different functions in your body:

Sodium controls fluid levels and aids nerve and muscle function.

Potassium supports heart, nerve, and muscle functions. It moves nutrients into cells and waste products out while supporting your metabolism.

Calcium helps blood vessels contract and expand to stabilize blood pressure. It secretes hormones and enzymes that help the nervous system send messages.

Chloride helps maintain healthy blood levels, blood pressure, and body fluids.

Magnesium aids nerve and muscle function and promotes the growth of healthy bones and teeth.

Phosphate supports the skeletal system, as well as nerve and muscle function.

Bicarbonate helps balance acids and basic alkaline compounds in blood (pH balance) and helps move carbon dioxide through your bloodstream.

THE FIVE DEFICIENCIES THE WESTERN WORLD GAVE YOU

Let's talk about what the modern lifestyle quietly steals from you.

If you live in the Western world — high stress, processed food, fluorescent lighting, and an inbox that never empties — there is a very good chance your body is running on empty in ways you haven't even identified yet. Not dramatically empty. Subtly empty. The kind of empty that shows up as brain fog, poor recovery, low energy, irritability, and a nagging sense that something just isn't quite right. The kind that no doctor's appointment seems to fix because nobody's actually looking for it.

Here are the five most common deficiencies. And the first thing I want you to understand is this — the best way to correct any of them isn't a pill. It's your plate.

Number one. Magnesium.

This one is the silent epidemic. Magnesium is involved in over three hundred biochemical reactions in your body. Sleep, muscle recovery, stress regulation, nerve function — magnesium is quietly running the show behind all of it. And most people in the West are chronically low because our soil has been stripped of it, and our stress hormones burn through what little we do absorb.

Before you reach for a supplement, reach for dark leafy

greens. Spinach, swiss chard, kale — load your plate. Pumpkin seeds are extraordinary — a small handful gives you a significant hit. Dark chocolate, avocado, black beans, almonds, cashews. These aren't exotic foods. They're real foods that your great-grandmother would have eaten without thinking twice.

If you do supplement, the form matters enormously. A blend of magnesium citrate, glycinate, threonate, and taurate gives you the broadest systemic coverage — each form targets different tissue. But food first. Always food first.

Number two. Iodine.

Your thyroid runs your metabolic engine. And your thyroid runs on iodine. When iodine is low, everything slows — metabolism, cognition, energy, mood. The Western diet replaced iodine-rich traditional foods with processed alternatives that actually block iodine absorption. That's not a conspiracy theory. That's chemistry.

The ocean has been providing humans with iodine since before civilization had a name for it. Seaweed — particularly kelp — is the single richest natural source on the planet. Coastal cultures that eat it regularly simply don't have thyroid problems at the rates we do. Wild-caught fish and shellfish are excellent sources. Oysters. Cod. Shrimp. Eggs from pasture-raised hens. These are your targets.

If you supplement, sea kelp in its natural form is the preferred route — your body recognizes it, absorbs it, and uses it the way nature intended.

Number three. Vitamin C.

Here's something that should stop you cold — humans are one of the only mammals on earth that cannot synthesize their own Vitamin C. Every other animal makes it internally. We have to eat it. Every single day. And under stress — physical, emotional, environmental — your body burns through it at a dramatic rate.

The good news is that whole foods make this one easy to solve. Bell peppers — especially the red ones — contain more Vitamin C than an orange. Kiwi, strawberries, papaya, broccoli, guava, kale. Eat these foods raw where possible. Heat destroys Vitamin C. A fresh salad does more for your immune system than a cooked meal of the same ingredients.

When supplementing, skip the cheap ascorbic acid tablets. Liposomal Vitamin C — particularly berry-based — is absorbed at a cellular level in a way that standard supplements simply cannot match. But again. Real food. Every day.

Number four. Sodium.

This one surprises people because we've been told for decades that sodium is the enemy. The truth is more precise than that — *processed* sodium, stripped of its mineral companions and dumped into packaged food, is problematic. But real, unprocessed sodium is essential. Your nerves run on it. Your muscles contract with it. Your hydration depends on it.

Celtic salt — harvested from the sea and dried by the sun — retains its full mineral profile. Eighty-plus trace minerals intact. Compare that to table salt, which has been refined down to two compounds and then had synthetic iodine added back in as an afterthought.

Your whole food sources here are straightforward: celery, beets, carrots, and artichokes contain natural sodium in balanced form. Olives. Fermented foods like kimchi and sauerkraut. Bone broth — which is essentially a mineral bath in a cup. Use real salt on real food. Your body will know the difference.

Number five. Vitamin E.

Vitamin E is a fat-soluble antioxidant — which means it protects your cells from oxidative damage. For athletes and high performers who train hard and generate significant metabolic stress, this one matters more than most people realize. Low Vitamin E contributes to muscle weakness, slow recovery, and immune suppression.

The food sources here are some of the most satisfying you'll eat. Sunflower seeds. Almonds. Hazelnuts. Wheat germ. Avocado — again. Spinach — again. Notice a pattern? The warrior's plate keeps looking the same. Dark greens, healthy fats, quality seeds and nuts. This is what traditional diets looked like before the food industry decided convenience mattered more than nutrition.

When supplementing, look for tocopherol — specifically mixed tocopherols. Avoid synthetic dl-alpha-tocopherol, which is the cheap version found in most store shelves and does more harm than good at high doses.

The common thread across all five of these is the same thread that runs through everything in this book. The answer isn't complicated. It isn't found in a pharmacy. It's found in returning — deliberately, stubbornly — to the foods that humans have eaten for thousands of years.

Dark greens. Quality proteins. Seeds and nuts. Ocean foods. Real salt. Fresh fruit eaten as nature packaged it.

Fill your plate with those things first. Then, if your lifestyle demands it, supplement intelligently with the forms your body can actually use.

But never let a pill replace a meal. The vessel deserves better than that.

Those of us in the Western world are also chronically low on micronutrients due to depleted soils— Common deficiencies include: copper, zinc, B vitamins, vitamin D, vitamin A, iron, potassium, niacin, folate, boron and selenium. Caution must be taken when supplementing these as it is possible to take toxic amounts, or create a deficiency of other nutrients.

Clinical trials indicate that a balanced intake of vitamins and minerals in natural form—or less ideally, as supplementation—helps your body repair at peak rates. In particular, gut health and the prevention of diverticulitis benefit significantly from vitamin C. Magnesium is seen as the wonder mineral, and vitamin C as the wonder vitamin, and their collective benefits cannot be overstated. Do not be afraid of proper real quality salt supplementation. But beware, regular non–iodized table salt is not salt only, often less than 30% pure, and is combined with glass and additives. Salt shaker at a restaurant table? Avoid.

Of course, this is a cursory overview and not in any way an exhaustive examination. Each of us should have tests at regular intervals to find out and address our specific needs.

Water: Key to High Performance

Your body is approximately 60% water. Your brain is 73% water. Your muscles are 79% water. Every metabolic process requires water. Dehydration of just 2% body weight measurably decreases performance, reaction time, and decision–making.

Yet most people walk around chronically dehydrated without realizing it. Thirst is a late indicator—by the time you feel thirsty, you're already dehydrated. For warriors, this is unacceptable.

The quality of water matters as much as quantity. Tap water in most Western cities contains chlorine, fluoride, pharmaceutical residues, heavy metals, and agricultural runoff. You wouldn't put contaminated oil in your car. Don't put contaminated water in your body.

Filter your water. At minimum, use a quality carbon filter that removes chlorine, volatile organic compounds, and common contaminants. Good: tested clean natural spring water. Better: reverse osmosis filtration that removes nearly everything, then re–mineralize with organic trace minerals. Best: distilled water (100% pure) supplemented with organically produced trace minerals sporadically.

Be careful about re-mineralizing water and scrutinize these products well. There are bio available minerals and non-bio available. If a vegetable or plant processes and outputs minerals in its leaves and fruit, you can utilize these organic minerals directly. Non-bio available minerals are about as good for your body as swallowing a handful of rocks and dirt and saying you ate minerals. Inorganic minerals pass through the body with little absorption and worse, can leach other minerals in the process, or at minimum cause your body stress trying to put them to waste. Both types of minerals are available for sale, make sure to get the bio-available.

Not just Clean Water

The containers matter too. Plastic bottles leach endocrine disruptors into water, especially when exposed to heat or stored long-term. BPA-free doesn't mean safe—BPS and other alternatives may be equally problematic.

Use glass or stainless steel containers. Store water away from sunlight and heat. If you must use plastic, never reuse single-use bottles and never let them get warm.

Water Quantities

How much water will you need? Basic formula: half your body weight in ounces daily, more if training hard or in hot conditions. A 200-pound athlete needs 100 ounces minimum, potentially 150+ on heavy training days. Water is best at room temperature. Ice cold water shocks the system and is not quickly absorbed.

Timing matters. Don't gulp water all at once. Sip consistently throughout the day. Front-load hydration—drink more in the morning and early afternoon, taper in the evening to avoid disrupting sleep with bathroom trips.

During training: Monitor hydration by checking urine color (pale yellow is ideal) and weighing yourself before and after sessions. For every pound lost, drink 16–20 ounces of water to re-hydrate properly.

Add electrolytes during intense or prolonged training. Water alone can dilute electrolyte concentrations. Use quality electrolyte supplements or make your own with Celtic salt, squeeze of lemon, and touch of raw honey.

Some advocate structured water or alkaline water. The results are mixed. What's proven: clean water in adequate amounts is foundational. Everything else is optimization once you've nailed the basics.

Cookware: Hidden Toxins in Your Kitchen

You pay attention to what you eat. But do you pay attention to what you cook it in?

Most conventional cookware leaches toxic compounds into your food. Non-stick coatings contain PFAS (forever chemicals) that accumulate in your body and disrupt hormones, thyroid function, and immune response. Even when cookware claims to be PFAS-free, the alternatives are often equally problematic.

Aluminum cookware leaches aluminum into acidic foods. Aluminum accumulation has been linked to neurological issues. Your brain doesn't need heavy metals.

Copper cookware can leach copper in excessive amounts, creating mineral imbalances and oxidative stress.

Teflon and non-stick coatings also release toxic fumes when overheated. Even at normal cooking temperatures, they degrade over time and flake into your food.

Safe alternatives:

Cast iron: The original non-stick when properly seasoned. Adds small amounts of beneficial iron to food. Lasts generations. Requires maintenance but worth it.

Stainless steel: Inert and non-reactive. Look for high-quality 18/10 stainless steel. Avoid cheap stainless that can leach nickel. Takes practice to prevent sticking but rewards skill.

Glass: Perfect for baking and storing. Completely inert. Breaks easily but causes no contamination.

Ceramic: True ceramic (not ceramic-coated) is safe and non-reactive. Make sure it's lead-free and from reputable manufacturers.

Carbon steel: Like cast iron but lighter. Requires seasoning. Excellent heat distribution. Professional chefs prefer it for good reason.

Avoid at all costs: Non-stick coatings, aluminum (unless anodized), copper (unless lined), cheap cookware from unknown manufacturers (often contains lead or cadmium).

The cookware you use every day either supports your health or slowly poisons you. Choose wisely.

Alcohol: The Performance Killer

Let's be direct: alcohol is poison. The dose makes it less lethal, but it's fundamentally a toxin you must process and eliminate. None is best, some feels like weakness and a lot is totally counterproductive. In my younger days, especially as a bouncer, I was guilty of enjoying the drink too much, and I know the harm it dealt against all my cardio work, nutrient load and bodies oxidative repair. I endorse marijuana as a substitute, if you insist on a substance to "take the edge off" from a long week.

Many fighters justify drinking as stress relief or celebration. Here's what actually happens:

Sleep disruption: Alcohol may help you fall asleep, but it destroys sleep quality. It suppresses REM sleep—the phase critical for memory consolidation, learning, and emotional regulation. You wake up less recovered, with elevated cortisol and compromised cognitive function.

Blood Thinning and blood pressure: Alcohol consumption

creates the conditions for high blood pressure due to constantly thin blood. Thin blood flows from cuts and knicks faster, blinding you if it is from a head wound ie: eye brow abrasion. The tunnel vision from high blood pressure limits peripheral awareness. Your BPM starts at a higher baseline, limiting the bodies ability to maintain stasis. All bad results for fighters trying to win.

Recovery impairment: Alcohol interferes with protein synthesis. It reduces human growth hormone secretion. It increases inflammation. A single night of drinking can set back recovery from training by days. It also blocks the uptake of vitamins and reduces the stomach acid needed to absorb B12.

Testosterone suppression: Alcohol lowers testosterone and raises estrogen. This affects muscle building, fat loss, lowers aggression, confidence, and sexual function.

Immune suppression: Alcohol compromises immune function for 24–48 hours after consumption. During heavy training when you're already immuno-suppressed, doubles the risk of illness.

Dehydration: Alcohol is a diuretic. It depletes electrolytes. It stresses the kidneys. Dehydration compounds all the other negative effects.

Cognitive impairment: Even small amounts slow reaction time, impair judgment, and reduce coordination for hours after consumption. You cannot afford this.

The data is unambiguous, alcohol consumption in any amount reduces athletic performance. The only debate is how much damage different doses cause.

Some argue red wine contains beneficial compounds like resveratrol. True. You can get resveratrol from grapes, berries, or supplements without the toxic effects of alcohol. Don't fool yourself.

If you're serious about performance, eliminate alcohol entirely. If you're not willing to do that, limit to rare occasions and understand you're choosing short-term pleasure over long-term excellence.

Warriors throughout history understood this. Many martial arts traditions forbid alcohol for practitioners. They weren't being moralistic—they recognized that sobriety is a calculated advantage.

When your opponent drinks and you don't, you've won before the fight starts. While they're recovering from weekend indulgence, you're training sharp and focused. The combined advantage compounds over months and years.

Alcohol was called "spirits" for a reason—it affects your spirit, your life force, your clarity. If you want to embody the warrior path, consider whether alcohol serves that goal or sabotages it.

Diet Fundamentals: What to Eat

What is the high octane fuel the performance athlete needs everyday? Raw, whole and organic (Non-GMO), with no sprays. The simplest, most complete, and nutritious foods in the most basic forms: meat, eggs, dairy, vegetables, fruits. You should be able to identify what the food is when you see it.

To get good food, you should stop eating what tastes the best.

The Western food industry has engineered products to hijack your taste buds and override your satiety signals. They've spent billions figuring out exactly what combinations of fat, salt, and sugar will make you crave more regardless of whether you need it. The very same scientists that designed cigarettes to be addictive, crafted the best selling processed foods for the big brand names.

Real food doesn't come in boxes with ingredient lists you can't pronounce. Real food spoils if you leave it out. Real food your great-grandmother would recognize.

Meal Rules:

1. Eat organic food with no sprays or chemicals.
2. Make meal time peaceful.
3. Chew your food fully.
4. During meals, if you must drink, sip only a little water.
5. Eat 20 calories per pound of body weight.
6. Eat 2 grams of protein per pound of body weight.
7. Rest 20 minutes after eating.

These are simple rules that you will reward you for following.

Brain Health and Cognitive Performance

Your brain is fat and water. We are surrounded daily with poisons : lead, mercury, air pollutants, paint fumes, synthetic cloths and bedding, microplastics, mold, pesticides, alcohol, chemical fragrances.

To maintain peak cognitive function—which directly impacts your ability to make split-second decisions in combat—you must protect your brain.

Protect the Command Center

Your brain is the most expensive real estate you own. Everything runs through it. Every decision, every reaction, every technique you've drilled ten thousand times — it all gets filtered through that three-pound organ sitting behind your eyes. And most people treat it like a rental property they have no intention of maintaining.

Let's fix that.

Sleep

Seven to eight hours. Not six and a half with a podcast on. Not five hours and a Red Bull chaser. Seven to eight, in a dark room, with your phone somewhere that isn't next to your head.

If you're consistently sleeping nine, ten, eleven hours and still waking up exhausted — that's not laziness. That's a signal. Sleep apnea, chronic infection, nutritional deficiency, unresolved stress load. Something is wrong and your body is burning through recovery bandwidth just trying to keep you functional. Don't ignore it. Investigate it.

Sleep is when your brain literally cleans itself. There's a waste clearance system — the glymphatic system — that only activates during deep sleep. It flushes out metabolic debris including the proteins associated with cognitive decline. You can't hack that with a supplement. You can't replace it with a nap. You just have to sleep. Properly. Consistently.

Toxins

This one people resist because it sounds fringe until you actually look at what's in your immediate environment.

Your bedding. Your air. Your water. Your cleaning products. Your synthetic fragrances that get sprayed, diffused, and washed into everything you own. The off-gassing from furniture built with particleboard and chemical adhesives. The mold quietly colonizing the corner of the bathroom nobody looks at.

Your brain is fat and water. It absorbs everything — including the things you'd rather not think about. Filter your water. Open your windows. Get natural fiber bedding — cotton, wool, linen. Stop spraying synthetic fragrance on your body and calling it grooming. These aren't radical lifestyle choices. They're basic maintenance on the most critical system you have.

Medication

Here's where I'll say something that was obvious up and until recent decades.

Your body was built to heal. Given real food, adequate sleep, and consistent movement, the human body has a staggering capacity for self-repair that modern medicine systematically underestimates because there is no profit margin in it.

Every pharmaceutical intervention carries a downstream cost. Side effects don't announce themselves loudly — they arrive quietly as new symptoms. And there is a well-worn clinical pathway where the prescription for the side effects of the first drug leads to a second drug, which creates a third problem, which leads to a third prescription. I've watched it happen to people who walked into a doctor's office with one complaint and walked out six months later managing a portfolio of medications like a failing investment.

That is not health care. That is symptom management at a profit.

Use medicine when you need it. Acute injury, genuine crisis, things your body genuinely cannot resolve without intervention — yes. Absolutely. But aspirin for a headache that eight glasses of water would solve? That's not treatment. That's avoidance. Find the root problem. Fix the root problem.

Fresh air

This one should be obvious and somehow isn't.

You were not designed for recirculated building air. The average office, apartment, or gym is a cocktail of dust, mold spores, volatile organic compounds, and whatever everyone else has been breathing and exhaling all day. Your lungs evolved processing air that moved, that carried oxygen from living plants, that changed with the weather.

Go outside. Every day. Not to your car. Outside. Walk around the block. Stand in it. Breathe like you mean it — slow, deep, through your nose, which is the filtration system your mouth isn't. Ten minutes of real air does something to your head that no amount of indoor productivity hacking can replicate. Spend time near water or trees if you can access either. This isn't poetry — it's physiology.

Caffeine

Black coffee before training — I'm with you entirely. The research on caffeine and athletic performance is about as solid as it gets. Focus sharpens, pain tolerance increases, output goes up. Use it deliberately and it earns its place.

But here's the distinction most people blur. There's a difference between using caffeine as a tool and using it as scaffolding. When the third cup of the day exists solely because you're too fatigued to function without it — you haven't solved a performance problem. You've pasted over a recovery problem. The fatigue is information. It's your body filing a formal complaint. Drowning it in stimulants doesn't answer the complaint. It just turns down the volume until the problem gets loud enough that caffeine can't cover it anymore.

Use it like you use every other tool in the arsenal. With intention. With restraint. And never as a substitute for fixing what's actually broken.

The brain is not separate from training. It is training. Take care of it like you take care of your joints, your conditioning, your technique. Because the day your body needs to perform at its absolute limit — you will need every part of that system firing clean.

Chemical Burdens We Carry

Be careful with chemicals and lotions, bug spray and sunscreen, detergents, soaps, and deodorant. Your skin is your largest organ. It absorbs everything you put on it directly into your bloodstream, bypassing some 's natural filtration systems.

Most commercial personal care products contain hormone disruptors, carcinogens, and neurotoxins. Parabens, phthalates, synthetic fragrances, triclosan, formaldehyde releasers—the list is extensive and disturbing.

Read labels. Choose products with ingredients you can pronounce. Better yet, use nothing your great-grandmother wouldn't recognize as safe to put on skin.

Sunscreen deserves special attention. You need sun exposure for vitamin D production and circadian rhythm regulation. Most sunscreens contain chemicals that act as endocrine disruptors. They're absorbed systemically and stored in fat tissue.

If you must use sunscreen, choose mineral-based (zinc oxide or titanium dioxide) rather than chemical sunscreens. Better: build a base tan gradually, wear protective clothing, and limit exposure during peak UV hours.

Bug spray containing DEET is a neurotoxin. It works, but at what cost? Natural alternatives using essential oils provide some protection. Better: avoid areas with heavy insect populations during peak times, wear protective clothing, use physical barriers like netting.

Deodorants containing aluminum have been linked to neurological issues and breast cancer. Aluminum blocks sweat glands—your body's natural detoxification system. Switch to aluminum-free alternatives or make your own with coconut oil, baking soda, and essential oils.

Detergents and soaps leave residues on your clothes and skin. You're in constant contact with these chemicals. Choose fragrance-free, dye-free options. Your skin will thank you.

Do not discount the cumulative effects of overworking your body's systems. Calculated awareness applied to the chemical warfare being waged by an industry that profits from your ignorance. Every chemical you avoid is one less stressor you must process and eliminate.

Ancient Wisdom, Modern Application

Chinese natural medicine, which could work in harmony with modern approaches, has, like all ancient nature-based wisdoms, sadly taken a back seat to profit-oriented and patent-holding synthetic pharmaceuticals.

Allopathic medicine excels at acute intervention—fixing broken bones, stopping infections, performing surgery. But for optimization, for prevention, for the daily maintenance of peak performance, traditional approaches often prove superior.

Seven thousand years of Chinese civilization developed dietary and herbal approaches based on observable results across countless generations. That sage wisdom shouldn't be dismissed simply because it doesn't fit the profit model of the pharmaceutical industry.

The principles of Chinese medicine—balancing hot and cold foods, eating seasonally, using food as medicine, understanding individual constitutions—have stood the test of time. They recognize that each person is unique and requires individualized approaches, not one-size-fits-all protocols.

Ayurveda from India, traditional Chinese medicine, Native American healing practices—these systems understood the interconnectedness of integrated self long before modern science began proving the mechanisms.

You don't have to choose one or the other. Take the best from all systems. Use modern testing to identify deficiencies and imbalances. Use traditional wisdom to address them through diet, herbs, and lifestyle. Use allopathic medicine when acute intervention is necessary.

The warrior path has always been about using every available tool. Don't limit yourself to one paradigm when multiple approaches offer value.

Dental Health

Your teeth are connected to meridians governing your extremities and vital organs. Ancient Asian cultures understood what Western medicine is only now rediscovering: the body functions as one integrated system. Energy, blood, and interstitial fluid flow through interconnected pathways—meaning any intervention that doesn't consider the whole body can do more harm than good. The mouth isn't separate from the body. It's a gateway.

Dental health impacts whole-body performance in profound ways. Root canals, mercury fillings, chronic infections—these create systemic inflammation that sabotages everything from cardiovascular function to immune response. Someone whom I respect, Dr. Hal Huggins, pioneered protocols recognizing these connections, and substantial research exists for those who want to dig deeper into the biological mechanisms at play.

Take care of your teeth. Find a holistic or naturopathic dentist who understands the whole-body implications of dental work—someone who treats the system, not just the symptom.

The point is simple: your dental health is your physical health. Treat it that way.

Meals for Battle: Fueling the Fight

Every preparation you've made — the drilling, the sparring, the early mornings, the weight cuts, the mental rehearsal — all of it can be undermined in the seventy-two hours before you compete if you treat nutrition as an afterthought. Most fighters train like professionals and eat like amateurs. Don't be that fighter.

Here's how you load the weapon.

Days Before

Starting two to three days out, carbohydrates become your primary job. Eight to twelve grams per kilogram of body weight per day. Your muscles have a fuel tank — glycogen — and right now your only concern is filling it to the top. Keep protein steady at two grams per kilogram. Fat stays low. This isn't the week for the fancy dinner or the cheat meal your training partner keeps suggesting. Tactical logistics. You're packing the vehicle for a long trip and every decision is about the journey ahead, not the pleasure of the moment.

Night Prior

Carbohydrates, moderate protein, fat kept to a minimum. Fat is slow — it sits in your gut like a houseguest that won't leave, and the last thing you want on fight morning is your digestive system still working on last night's meal. Keep it simple. Keep it familiar. A meal you've eaten a hundred times. Your nervous system is already running hot with anticipation — it's not the moment to introduce a variable.

Eat early enough that you go to bed with digestion mostly done and sleep as your body's final preparation.

Fight Morning

Three to four hours out. Light. Carbohydrate-based. Toast with honey. A bowl of oatmeal. Banana and rice. Nothing exotic, nothing experimental, nothing your training partner swears by but you've never actually tried. Fight day is not a testing ground. Everything on your plate today has already been proven in training. The only thing being tested today is your opponent.

One Hour Out

If you need it — and some people don't — a small hit of simple carbohydrates. A piece of fruit. An energy gel. A few sips of a sports drink. The keyword is small. Your digestive system needs to be quiet when the bell rings, not working. At this point you're topping off the tank, not filling it. There's a difference.

During — (if the event runs long)

For anything lasting beyond sixty to ninety minutes, your glycogen stores will begin to deplete in ways that become performance-limiting. Thirty to sixty grams of carbohydrates per hour through sports drinks or gels keeps the engine fed. Think of it as pit stops. Formula One teams don't guess about fuel. Neither should you.

After

This window gets wasted more than any other. The fight is done, the adrenaline is still moving through you, your mind is already replaying every exchange — and your muscles are sitting there with the door wide open, primed to absorb everything you give them for repair and rebuilding. Miss this window and you've extended your recovery by days.

Carbohydrates and protein in roughly a two-to-one ratio within thirty minutes of finishing. Chocolate milk — genuinely one of the most effective recovery drinks ever studied and one of the cheapest. A protein shake with a banana. A recovery drink. Whatever it is, get it in while the window is open.

Your body runs on ATP — adenosine triphosphate — the actual energy currency your cells trade in. Every punch thrown, every level change, every explosive scramble on the ground draws from that account. Nutrition timing is how you make sure the account never runs dry at the moment you can least afford it.

You trained too hard to lose because you ate wrong. That would be an inexcusable way to leave performance on the table — and unlike your opponent, your lunch is entirely within your control.

Advanced Optimization: Beyond the Basics

Once you've mastered the fundamentals—clean food, proper timing, adequate hydration, quality sleep—there are advanced interventions worth considering:

a) Vitamin C injection: Intravenous vitamin C bypasses digestive limitations and achieves blood concentrations impossible through oral supplementation. Some athletes use this pre–competition for immune support and as an antioxidant to combat oxidative stress from intense training. Obviously this requires qualified medical supervision.

b) Oxygen therapy: Hyperbaric oxygen chambers increase oxygen dissolved in blood plasma, potentially enhancing recovery and healing. Elite athletes and military special operations use this. Expensive but effective for specific applications.

c) Blood work regularly: [Test, don't guess.] Comprehensive panels revealing vitamin levels, hormone profiles, inflammatory markers, and metabolic function allow precise interventions rather than blanket supplementation.

d) Mitochondrial support: Your mitochondria are cellular power plants. Support them with CoQ10, PQQ, R+alpha–lipoic acid, and L–carnitine. As you age, mitochondrial function declines. Supplementation can partially offset this.

e) Managing inflammation: Chronic inflammation destroys performance and health. Beyond diet, consider curcumin (with black pepper for absorption), omega–3 fatty acids from fish oil, and addressing iron overload if relevant. Some inflammation is necessary for adaptation. Too much prevents recovery.

g) Trigger point and Plasma Injections: I did these every two weeks for a year. Mixed reviews from me.

f) Stem Cells. I have had several treatments over the years, including epidural shots that included hip operations to harvest my own marrow cells. Each surgery was completed over two days. The IV general therapy we sourced stem cells from adipose fat and blood platelets spun down to irrigate the areas around my spinal L5/S1 injuries. I am fully recovered from damaged discs. I had great experiences here.

Brain–healthy supplements based on naturopathic research:

- Lion's mane mushroom for brain growth and nerve repair
- L–theanine for calming focus

- Acetyl L-carnitine for brain function
- Rhodiola rosea for stress relief
- Ginkgo biloba for memory and circulation
- Royal jelly for clarity and hormone balance
- Citicoline for brain cell membrane growth
- Bacopa monnieri for memory recall and speed

There are newer and more advanced tools, I recommend using doctors from large city sports team franchises, a great sports doctor is worth their weight in gold.

Garbage Out – Reading the Results

It stands to reason that if you do everything right from diet choices, proper preparation and intake timing, quality water, good sleep, no poisons, drugs or alcohol, you should be good right? Well, test and verify. Blood tests will tell a lot, hair samples, retina scans, and yes the toilet. Run urinalysis for PH and glucose, ketones and more. Check color, quantity and flow. Examine stool for color, shape, consistency, size and timing. It is a cheap and easy way to gauge if you are on the right track. Consultation with your health professional will help you to set a baseline and monitor changes.

Bottom Line

With health, you have a thousand hopes. Without it, you have but one.

Your body is the vehicle through which you experience life and accomplish every goal. Feed it properly. Time your nutrition strategically. Cultivate your gut microbiome. Respect your circadian rhythms. Minimize toxic exposure. Supplement intelligently based on your individual needs. Hydrate consistently with clean water. Eliminate alcohol. Avoid chemical burden from personal care products and cookware.

Garbage in, garbage out. The inverse is equally true: quality in, excellence out.

The fight is won or lost long before you step into the ring. It's won in the kitchen, in the choices you make three times a day, every day, for years. The combined advantage of proper nutrition compounds over time into measurable performance differences.

Your opponent might train as hard. They might be as technically skilled. But if they fuel their body like a dumpster while you fuel yours like a Formula 1 race car, the outcome is predetermined.

Respect the body you've been given. Feed it like your life depends on it.

Because it does.

CHAPTER 9 – TIMING RECOVERY

"The pain you feel today, is the strength you feel tomorrow."—Stephan Richards. 2017

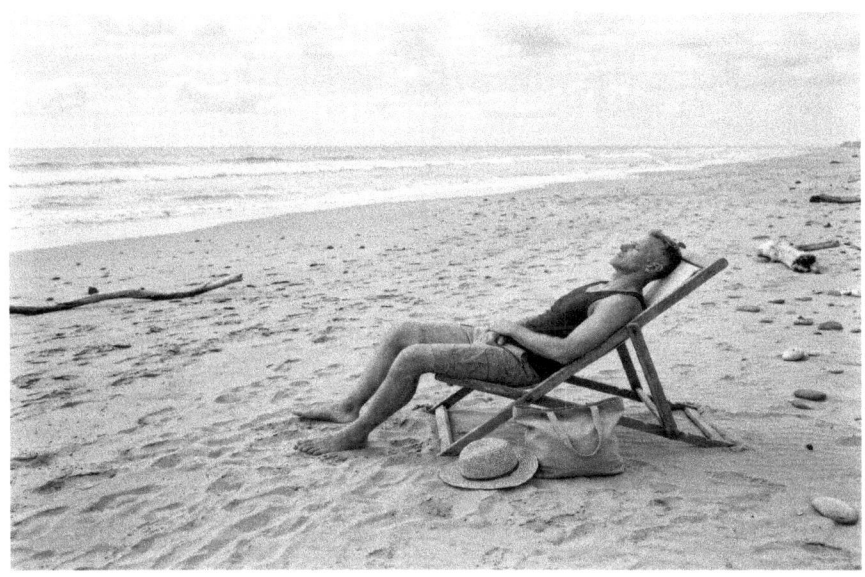

Optimizing Your Circadian Rhythm: Warrior's Clock

Your body operates on a 24–hour cycle that has been hardwired into your biology over many hundreds of generations. This circadian rhythm isn't just about when you feel sleepy—it's a sophisticated system that regulates every aspect of your comprehensive performance. Understanding and respecting this natural clock is the difference between training smart and training stupid.

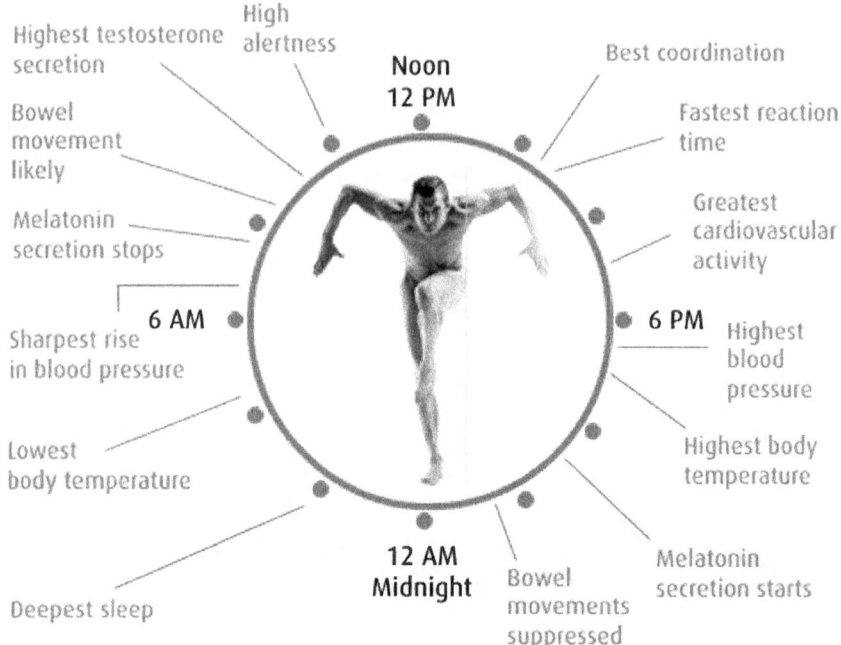

Referring to the graphic, higher work-rates (power output or effort level) are best timed for the early evening. Individual differences in performance rhythms are small but significant. Circadian rhythms are larger in amplitude in physically fit individuals than sedentary individuals. Athletes over 50 years of age tend to be higher in "morningness," and they habitually schedule more training earlier in the morning and generally injecting more intensity during exercise compared with young athletes.

Consider what happens throughout your day. At 6 AM, your blood pressure rises sharply and melatonin secretion stops—your body is literally waking itself up at the hormonal level. This is followed by your highest testosterone secretion and the likelihood of bowel movement, preparing you for the day ahead. By noon, you're at peak alertness. Your body knows this is prime time for cognitive work and complex decision-making. At 6 PM, your cardiovascular activity peaks along with your blood pressure and temperature. Your body is primed for maximum physical output—the ideal training window for explosive power and strength work.

As evening approaches, melatonin secretion begins around 9 PM, signaling your body to start winding down. By midnight, you hit your deepest sleep, and by 6 AM, your temperature drops to its lowest point—when your body does its deepest recovery work. Then the cycle repeats.

Circadian variations in sports performance shows that peak performance time of day is around 6 PM. The majority of components of sports performance—flexibility, muscle strength, short-term high-power output—vary with time of day in a sinusoidal manner and peak in the early evening close to the daily maximum in temperature.

Learn to work with the body, to understand the optimum timing for tasks and rest. The circadian cycle, matched with appropriate sunlight exposure both at sunrise and sunset, can heal and balance the body.

Female Training Cycle

For females ages 13–45, the 24-hour circadian cycle operates within a second, overlapping rhythm: the approximately 28-day menstrual or infradian cycle. These two cycles interact to create windows of enhanced or reduced training capacity. Condensing this to the key elements; The follicular phase (approx. days 4–14, just after menstruation begins), when estrogen rises, females experience optimal conditions for building muscle, power, and learning new motor skills. This phase pairs well with the evening circadian peak for maximum training adaptation. The mid-cycle ovulatory phase offers peak reaction time and explosive power. However, during the luteal phase (days 15–28), when progesterone dominates, recovery takes longer, temperature runs slightly higher (which can shift the circadian performance peak earlier), and injury risk increases. Rather than fighting these natural rhythms, strategic training respects both cycles: schedule intense skill work, strength training, and competition preparation during the follicular phase while emphasizing technique refinement, moderate-intensity work, and mobility during the luteal phase. Track both cycles to identify your personal patterns—the young martial artist who learns to surf these dual rhythms rather than ignore them gains a significant advantage in both performance and injury prevention.

All Athletes

To design the high-performance athlete, we need lots of sleep—a minimum of eight hours is vital. We should follow our metabolic guideline of operating in regular daytime hours and sleeping during geographical night. Miss this, and cognitive function dives.

We need to eat healthy, low-fat foods only in daylight hours, because fatty foods tend to have elements which turn off our internal programming to tell us when we're full. We should train during our peak performance times and get a nap in often. Do these things and you will be leaner, smarter, and happier.

Earthing and Grounding

Your body accumulates positive electrical charge through daily exposure to electronics, synthetic materials, and modern environments. This buildup disrupts your bioelectrical system, contributing to inflammation, poor sleep, and delayed recovery. The solution is ancient and free: direct contact with the earth. Being on the ground with no shoes allows excess positive charge to flow out and into the earth, while drawing negative ions back in—restoring a healthy electrical balance in your internal systems. In the health community it is called grounding or earthing. Walk barefoot on grass, dirt, sand, or concrete. Stand in contact with the earth for 20–30 minutes daily. Your nervous system will calm, inflammation will decrease, and recovery will accelerate. The earth is a massive reservoir of electrons. Use it.

Ride the Rhythm

Here's what most athletes get catastrophically wrong: they fight this rhythm instead of working with it. They stay up late staring at screens, flooding their system with blue light that suppresses melatonin production. They train at random times based on convenience rather than biological readiness. They eat heavy meals when their digestive system is trying to shut down for the night. They wonder why they're not making progress when they're literally sabotaging their body's natural optimization system.

A change to night shift or long distance travel for competitions can wreak havoc on the bodies internal clock. The normal circadian rhythms can be desynchronized following a flight across several time zones or a transfer to nocturnal operations. Although athletes show all the symptoms of jet lag—increased fatigue, disturbed sleep and circadian rhythms—performance effects depend on direction of travel, time of day of competition, and the various performance components involved in a particular sport. Arriving to your destination with sufficient lead time for your body to adjust to different climates, altitudes and time zones is wise. Rest and adequate recovery applies to any type of exertion, including travel. For adequately adjusted nighttime function, expect 10 days to a month for the average person to feel semi-normal again.

Circadian Rhythms and Performance

The warrior who respects the circadian rhythm structures their entire day around these biological peaks and valleys. They wake early when testosterone is highest—your body's signal to tackle the hardest comprehensive challenges of the day. They schedule their most intense training sessions between 3 PM and 6 PM when reaction time is fastest, cardiovascular output is highest, and temperature is optimal for performance. They understand that training at 10 PM might fit their schedule, but it's fighting against every biological signal their body is sending about rest and recovery.

Your deepest sleep happens between midnight and 6 AM. It is when growth hormone is released, when muscle tissue repairs, when your nervous system recovers from the day's training stress. If you're awake during these hours, you're not just losing sleep—you're losing the recovery that makes tomorrow's training possible. The fighter who sleeps from 10 PM to 6 AM will always outperform the fighter who sleeps from 2 AM to 10 AM, even if they get the same number of hours. It's not about duration alone—it's about alignment with your biological programming.

Consider what happens when you ignore this rhythm consistently. Your testosterone secretion gets disrupted. Your blood pressure regulation becomes erratic. Your temperature doesn't peak when it should. Your melatonin production gets confused. You're essentially putting your body in a constant state of jet lag, and you expect to perform at elite levels? It doesn't work. The body doesn't negotiate with your schedule—you negotiate with its requirements.

The practical application is simple but requires discipline. Go to bed at the same time every night, ideally before 10 PM. Wake at the same time every morning, no later than 6 AM. Eat your largest meals during the day when digestion is optimal. Schedule your hardest training when your body is primed for it—late afternoon for power and strength, morning for skill work and technique when your alertness is high but your body isn't fatigued. Avoid screens and bright lights after sunset. Let your melatonin rise naturally.

By optimizing your body's rhythm, you can be a finely-tuned machine. You can fight it and stay mediocre, or you can work with it and become exceptional. The circadian rhythm is a gift—it tells you exactly when to push, when to rest, when to eat, when to sleep. You decide what level of tune you want to run in.

The warrior who masters their internal clock masters their training. The warrior who ignores it wonders why they're always tired, always injured, always plateauing. Your body is giving you the blueprint for optimal performance every single day. Stop fighting it. Start following it. Align your life with your biology and watch what becomes possible.

Enlightened Rhythm

Early in the day, get direct sunlight in your eyes for 10–20 minutes. Taking in light without the filters of sunglasses and window glass panes will release hormones in your endocrine system to set your body up for waking up and tackling the day, or slowing down and going to sleep. These are the connections between you and the realm to which you are inexorably tied—an ally in keeping your body operating at its best.

It ain't just hippie wisdom—it triggers your cortisol awakening response, which sets your entire circadian clock for the day. Studies show this single habit:

- Advances the evening melatonin pulse by 1–2 hours
- Increases deep sleep duration (where growth hormone peaks)
- Improves testosterone production
- Enhances mitochondrial function in muscle tissue

Cloudy day? You need longer exposure (20–30 min). Artificial light doesn't cut it—you need the blue light spectrum at the intensity only the sun provides.

Evening: Heat exposure 90 minutes before bed

Have a hot bath, sauna, or hot shower (20 minutes at 104–107°F) approximately 90 minutes before sleep. Here's the paradox: heating your body triggers peripheral vasodilation—blood rushes to your extremities, which actually *cools your core temperature*. This mimics and enhances your natural circadian temperature drop that signals sleep onset.

Research shows:
a) Increases deep sleep by 10–15%
b) Accelerates sleep onset by 10 minutes
c) Elevates growth hormone secretion during sleep
d) Reduces inflammatory markers (IL–6, TNF–alpha)

Lesser-Known Addition: Non-Sleep Deep Rest (NSDR)

10–30 minute NSDR/Yoga Nidra sessions during the day (especially if sleep-deprived) can partially restore the neurochemical benefits of sleep and accelerate recovery. This enhances dopamine reserves by 60% and improves motor learning consolidation.

The warrior's edge: Most athletes focus only on *duration* of sleep. The real secret is optimizing *circadian amplitude*—the contrast between your daytime and nighttime states. Maximum light exposure early + complete darkness at night + temperature manipulation = compressed recovery windows.

Recovery: The Weapon Everyone Ignores

Most fighters think training is what makes them better. They're half right. Training is the stimulus that breaks you down. Recovery is what builds you back up stronger. If you're training hard but recovering poorly, you're just accumulating damage without adaptation. You're getting worse, not better, and you're too stupid or too stubborn to see it until you're injured or burned out.

Here's the truth that separates champions from pretenders: your body doesn't improve during training—it improves during recovery. When you push hard in the gym, you're creating micro-tears in muscle tissue, depleting energy stores, stressing your nervous system, and accumulating metabolic waste. That's necessary. That's the signal you need to adapt. But the actual adaptation—the muscle growth, the neural pathway reinforcement, the cardiovascular improvements—all of that happens when you're resting. If you never give your body time and resources to complete that process, you're just breaking yourself down without building anything back up.

Sleep is the foundation of all recovery. If you're sleeping less than seven hours a night, you're training at half capacity and you don't even know it. During deep sleep, your body releases growth hormone, repairs damaged tissue, consolidates motor learning from your training sessions, and clears metabolic waste from your brain. Miss this window and you're starting the next day with yesterday's damage still amassed. Do that for weeks or months and you're walking around in a perpetual state of half-broken.

But sleep alone isn't enough. Active recovery matters. Light movement, stretching, mobility work—these aren't just feel-good activities, they're critical for maintaining the systems that keep you training. Blood flow delivers nutrients to damaged tissue and removes waste products. If you train hard then sit on the couch for three days, your recovery slows to a crawl. The warrior moves every day, even on rest days. Not hard training—movement. Walk, stretch, swim, do yoga. Keep the systems flowing.

Nutrition is recovery fuel. You can't build muscle without protein. You can't replenish glycogen stores without carbohydrates. You can't regulate hormones without healthy fats. You can't do any of it without adequate calories. The fighter who trains six days a week but eats like a teenager is working against himself. you need building blocks to rebuild what training broke down. Give it chicken nuggets, pop and chips and you are going backwards fast.

Hydration and Recovery Cycles

Your body's repair systems run on water. During sleep, your cells flush metabolic waste, synthesize proteins for muscle repair, and regulate hormones that govern recovery—all processes requiring optimal hydration. Dehydration disrupts sleep architecture, reducing deep sleep phases where growth hormone peaks and tissue regeneration occurs most efficiently.

Your circadian rhythm depends on proper fluid balance. Dehydration triggers cortisol release at inappropriate times, throwing off your natural wake–sleep cycle and keeping you wired when you should be recovering. It also impairs the glymphatic system—your brain's waste removal process that operates primarily during deep sleep. Without adequate hydration, metabolic debris accumulates, cognitive function suffers, and morning recovery is incomplete.

Time your water intake strategically. Front-load hydration during daylight hours when your kidneys process fluids most efficiently. Taper intake two hours before bed to avoid disrupting sleep with bathroom breaks. Wake up, drink immediately—your body just spent eight hours without water and needs to rehydrate before anything else.

Clear or pale yellow urine throughout the day indicates proper hydration. Dark urine means your recovery is already compromised. Water isn't optional for warriors—it's the foundation of every regenerative process your body performs while you sleep.

Elite Plan for Recovery

Here's what separates elite athletes from good ones: the

elite treat recovery with the same intensity they treat training. They prioritize sleep like it's part of the workout. They schedule rest days and honor them. They eat to fuel performance and recovery, not just to satisfy hunger. They do their mobility work even when they don't feel like it. They get massages, ice baths, saunas—whatever tools accelerate the recovery process. They understand that recovery isn't passive rest, it's active restoration.

The average fighter trains hard and hopes for the best. The intelligent fighter trains hard and recovers harder. They understand that the training session ends when they leave the gym, but the work of becoming better continues for the next 23 hours. Every decision they make either supports recovery or undermines it. Sleep or stay up late? Eat clean or eat convenient? Move or be sedentary? Each choice compounds over time.

And here's the part most people miss: recovery isn't just physical. Your nervous system needs recovery. Your mental energy needs recovery. If you're constantly stressed, constantly stimulated, constantly grinding without ever downshifting—your body stays in sympathetic nervous system dominance. Fight or flight, all the time. That's not sustainable. You need parasympathetic activation—rest and digest mode—to allow deep recovery. That means meditation, breathwork, time in nature, activities that calm your nervous system rather than rev it up.

Avoiding fatigue and injury is just as valuable as quality work-outs. Listen to your body. If you're perpetually sore, perpetually tired, perpetually irritable—you're under-recovered. If your performance is plateauing or declining despite consistent training—you're under-recovered. If you're getting sick frequently, if minor injuries are becoming major ones, if your motivation is tanking—you're under-recovered. These are signals, not weaknesses. Your body is telling you it needs time and resources to rebuild. Ignoring these signals doesn't make you tough, it makes you stupid.

The warrior who masters recovery will always outlast the warrior who only masters training. Hard work is necessary but insufficient. Smart work—training hard when it's time to train, recovering hard when it's time to recover—that's the formula for long-term elite performance. You can't beat yourself into greatness. You have to build yourself into it, and building requires both the breakdown of training and the restoration during recovery.

Recovery is not weakness. Recovery is strategy. Recovery is how you stay in the fight for decades instead of burning out in years. Treat it with respect. Give it the time and attention it deserves. Because the fighter who can train hard today, recover completely, and train hard again tomorrow will always beat the fighter who trains hard today, barely recovers, and limps through tomorrow's session at 60% capacity.

Your body is not your enemy. It's your weapon. Take care of your weapon or it will fail you when you need it most.

CHAPTER 10 – SHARPEN THE MIND

"Perceive that which cannot be seen with the eye."—
Miyamoto Musashi, A Book of Five Rings, 1645

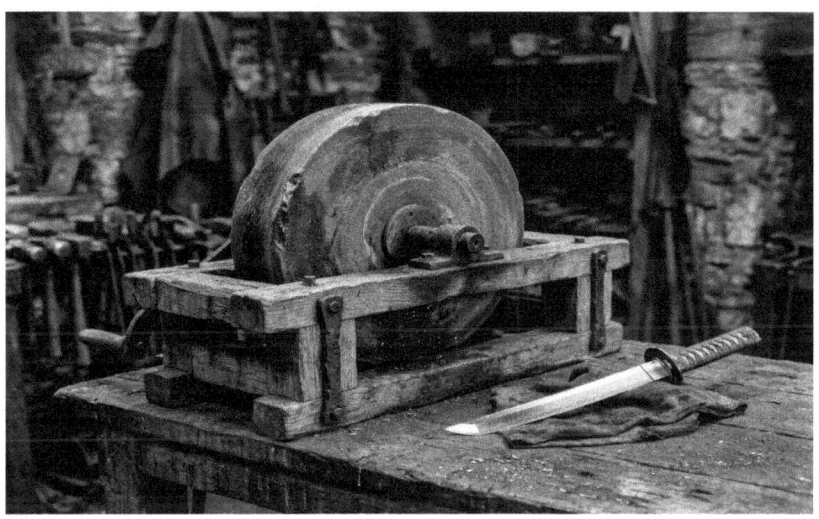

Our greatest weapon is our mind. I would much rather face a young, dumb muscleman than a devious old person. Why? Because strength fades, but strategy endures. The muscleman relies on physical dominance—predictable, finite, trainable against. The intelligent opponent sees three moves ahead. They identify your weaknesses before you know you have them. They set traps. They manipulate distance, timing, and psychology. They win before the fight begins.

Training the mind isn't optional—it's what separates competent fighters from true masters. Physical prowess gets you in the door. Mental acuity keeps you alive. You can drill techniques until your body moves on autopilot, but without the strategic mind to deploy them effectively, you're just a well-trained robot waiting to be outmaneuvered. The question isn't whether you're strong or skilled. **The question is: can you think under pressure?**

And thinking under pressure starts with how you train your perspective. Train to see opportunities, not obstacles. Re-imagine all of your actions as a game to win and excel at. Life is all about attitude and perspective. Your mind wants what's best for you—train to give it the tools and experiences to advise you quickly with accurate, intelligent decisions for winning results.

Intelligent decisions require intelligent awareness. I cannot stress this enough, always be aware of your surroundings. We're told to have our head on a swivel or to have eyes in the back of our head—euphemisms for being hyper-vigilant and hyper-aware of the proximal environment. Calculating the components and actors around you gives you an advantage as you assess potential outcomes based on active factors. But awareness alone isn't enough. **You can notice everything and still respond like an idiot.** You need the cognitive capacity to process what you observe and respond appropriately.

So what does intelligence actually mean for the martial artist?

Physical Wisdom

Intelligence can be described as the sum of the following traits and specific abilities and the speed at which they are employed in new, unique scenarios and environments:

Adaptability – A grappler who only knows ground fighting gets neutralized by an opponent who maintains distance. The intelligent martial artist cross-trains, practices multiple ranges, and develops versatility. Adaptability also means recognizing when your primary strategy isn't working and shifting approaches mid-fight.

Acquisition of Knowledge – It's not just passive absorption—it's active hunting for information. Study your opponent before you face them. Watch how they move. Identify patterns. Learn from every sparring session, every loss, every technique that catches you off guard. The intelligent fighter treats every experience as data.

Ability to Reason – During a fight, you're constantly solving problems: "He drops his left hand after throwing the jab. If I time a counter right, I can exploit that." Highest cognition and real-time reasoning under stress. Training develops this through progressive problem-solving—situational drills, conditional sparring, strategic games.

Percentage of Successful Outcomes – Intelligence isn't just thinking well—it's thinking effectively. You can have brilliant strategies that fail in execution. The intelligent martial artist tracks what actually works for them, abandons techniques that don't serve their body type or style, and doubles down on high-percentage moves.

Evaluations and Judgment – Can you accurately assess threat levels? Can you judge distance, timing, and when to commit to a technique? Poor judgment gets you hurt. Sound judgment keeps you safe while creating opportunities.

Original Productive Thought – Cookie-cutter techniques work until they don't. The intelligent martial artist innovates—adapts techniques to their unique attributes, creates combinations their opponents haven't seen, solves problems creatively. Bruce Lee didn't just learn—he synthesized and created.

Mental Acuity – Sharpness of mind. Processing speed. The fighter who sees the opening a half-second faster lands the strike. The fighter whose mind is sharp recognizes the feint before committing to the counter. This can be trained through deliberate practice using the exercises and we'll cover some methods later in this chapter.

These seven components don't operate independently—they compound. The fighter with strong adaptability AND high acquisition of knowledge makes better real-time decisions than either trait alone could produce. Together, they create the foundation upon which fighters wisdom is built.

Wisdom: Experience Applied

Wisdom is the collective historical understanding of past experience and the ability to employ lessons learned to new variations of similar problems. The more experiences you've had and remembered, the more lessons you can apply simultaneously to complex problems—creating an exponential effect that dramatically increases your chances of positive outcomes.

Here's how this works in combat: A white belt faces a jab for the first time and freezes. A blue belt recognizes the jab and executes their trained defense. A black belt sees the jab coming, recognizes the weight distribution that precedes it, identifies the likely follow-up based on the opponent's stance, and is already positioning for a counter before the punch is fully extended.

That's fighters wisdom—pattern recognition built from thousands of repetitions across hundreds of variations. The black belt isn't just responding to what's happening. They're drawing on combined experience to predict what will happen next and position themselves advantageously.

Wisdom in martial arts means:
- Learning from your losses more than your wins
- Recognizing when an instructor's correction echoes

something you learned years ago but finally understand now
- Connecting insights from different martial arts to create deeper understanding
- Knowing which techniques work in which contexts and why
- Understanding the difference between what looks effective and what is effective

This requires being able to analyze and interpret while responding appropriately, keeping calm, and applying solutions based on critical thinking and stored knowledge. It's not just about having the data—it's about accessing the right data at the right moment under pressure.

Knowledge Acquisition: Building Your Database

Knowledge and the ability to access it is a wonder of the human brain. Storing knowledge is a daily task, and with dedication, all of your spare moments can be advancing your information base. Reading and studying topics that support your areas of interest has large knock-on effects.

For example: Understanding muscle fiber types explains why some people excel at explosive power while others dominate in endurance. Knowing this helps you train to your strengths while addressing your weaknesses. Understanding leverage and biomechanics reveals why a smaller person can throw a larger opponent—it's not magic, it's physics applied through technique.

Knowledge of nutrition tells you why you gas out in the third round—maybe it's not conditioning, maybe it's fueling. Understanding inflammation and recovery explains why some training soreness is productive while other pain signals actual injury, and you need to back off and recover.

The martial artist who studies psychology understands fear responses, which helps in both managing their own fear and recognizing fear-based reactions in opponents. The martial artist who studies history learns from warriors across centuries and cultures, gaining insights that pure training can't provide.

This knowledge compounds. Each piece connects to others. Biomechanics connects to physics. Psychology connects to strategy. Nutrition connects to performance. The more comprehensive your knowledge base, the more connections you can make, and the more effective your training becomes.

Make learning systematic. Dedicate 30 minutes daily to study. Keep a training journal where you record not just physical progress but intellectual insights. When you learn something valuable, test it. Does it work in practice? Does it improve your performance? Knowledge without application is trivia.

Study biomechanics and sports sciences to understand how force transfers through the body. Study psychology to understand fear, aggression, and decision-making under stress. Study history to learn from warriors across cultures and centuries. Study philosophy to develop the ethical grounding that governs when and how you use your skills.

Read voraciously. Not just martial arts books—expand into adjacent fields. Neuroscience. Physics. Military strategy. Corporate leadership. Conflict resolution. Each discipline offers insights that enhance your martial practice.

Building Mental Capacity

As with every muscle in your body, if you exercise it, it will grow; if you don't use it, you lose it. Your mind is your most important muscle. It creates reality from thought. If you think it, you can take an idea and bring its fruits into the physical realm. Something from nothing. Here is the power of training —turning abstract concepts into concrete results through disciplined thought and action.

Mental Expansion: Cross-Training the Brain

Learning a second language, musical instruments, games like chess, or high-level mathematics—these are new ways to communicate and interact with challenge. Each expands your mind, gives you new perspectives, connects new synapses, and benefits your martial tools and tactics.

Why does learning a language make you a better fighter? Because language learning requires pattern recognition, memory, and the ability to operate within rule systems—the same skills needed to learn and execute martial arts techniques. Your brain doesn't compartmentalize as much as you think. Neural pathways built through language learning strengthen the same cognitive infrastructure used in combat.

Chess teaches you to think several moves ahead, to recognize patterns, to manage time pressure, to adapt when your strategy fails. These aren't just chess skills—they're fighting skills applied to a different domain. The chess grandmaster and the master martial artist share more cognitive similarities than differences.

Music develops timing, rhythm, and the ability to execute complex sequences automatically—essential skills for combining techniques into flowing combinations. Musicians understand the difference between practicing slowly with intention and performing at speed, which is exactly how martial arts training should progress.

Mathematics strengthens logical reasoning and problem-solving under constraint. Every fight is a math problem: angles, distance, timing, energy expenditure. The martial artist with strong mathematical thinking naturally calculates better than those who rely purely on instinct.

Each of these pursuits builds cognitive capacity that transfers to martial performance. You're not just becoming more well-rounded—you're building a more capable fighting brain.

Fueling the Mind

Your brain is the most expensive real estate in your body. It occupies 2% weight but consumes 20% of your total energy. It's the command center for every decision, every reaction, every technique you execute under pressure.

Your brain runs primarily on glucose, but not all glucose is created equal. The source matters. The timing matters. The consistency matters. Feed it garbage, and it performs like garbage. Feed it strategically, and you gain edges your opponents don't even know exist.

Simple carbohydrates—sugar, processed foods, energy drinks—spike blood glucose rapidly, creating a brief surge followed by a crash. Your brain experiences this as mental fog, impaired decision-making, and reduced reaction time. Complex carbohydrates from whole foods—vegetables, fruits, whole grains, legumes—provide steady glucose release that sustains mental performance throughout training.

Healthy fats—particularly omega-3 fatty acids from fish, nuts, and seeds—are crucial for neural function and the anti-inflammatory processes that protect your brain during intense training. Protein provides the amino acids necessary for neurotransmitter production—the chemical messengers that determine how quickly and accurately your brain processes information.

Hydration is equally critical. Even mild dehydration impairs cognitive function, slowing reaction time and dulling mental sharpness. If you're training hard and not drinking water consistently, you're operating in a compromised state mentally before you're compromised physically.

Guarding Your Thoughts

Your internal dialogue shapes your reality more than any external circumstance.

Negative self-talk isn't just demotivating—it's neurologically destructive. Every time you tell yourself "I can't do this" or "I'm not good enough," you're reinforcing neural pathways that make failure more likely. Your brain doesn't distinguish between external threats and self-generated negativity. Both trigger the same stress response that impairs performance.

This doesn't mean toxic positivity or denying reality. It means disciplined re-framing.

Instead of "I'll never be as good as that black belt," try "I'm not there yet, but every session closes the gap." Instead of "I got destroyed in sparring today," try "I identified three specific weaknesses to work on."

The technique: when you catch yourself in negative thought patterns, interrupt immediately. Say "stop" out loud if necessary. Then deliberately reframe. It may not be comfortable at first—but neither was your first day of training. discipline requires the same repetition as technique.

Guard your mind as vigilantly as you guard your face in sparring. Negative thoughts slip through your defense and land internal damage that accumulates over time. Do not think or dwell on the negative. The discipline you build through training extends beyond physical techniques—it shapes how you think, process conflict, and approach confrontation.

Taking Control: Locus of Control

Henry Ford said it perfectly: "Whether you think you can or you think you can't—you're right."

He wasn't pushing motivational fluff. It's actually neurological fact. Your beliefs about control determine whether you exercise it. Psychologists call this your **locus of control**—internal or external.

Internal locus: "I control my training, my diet, my preparation. My outcomes reflect my choices."

External locus: "My genetics are bad. My schedule is too busy. I'm too old to start. The worst always happens to me."

The difference determines your outcome. A martial artist with internal locus of control takes responsibility for their development. When they fail, they analyze what they can change. When they succeed, they understand what worked and replicate it. They see obstacles as problems to solve, not excuses for inaction.

A martial artist with external locus of control blames circumstances. They attribute success to luck and failure to factors beyond their control. This mindset is poison because it removes agency—and without agency, there is no growth.

Here's the trap most people fall into: mistaking permission for freedom. In the Western world, being an adult means you can have alcohol and pizza anytime you want. That's not freedom—that's marketing.

Real freedom is understanding the risk–reward trade-off and choosing what serves your goals over what satisfies immediate impulses. It's the ability to choose between right and wrong. But you can't exercise that freedom if you've been conditioned to believe the destructive choice *is* freedom. That's the perversion.

A disciplined mind pauses, recognizes there's a choice to make, and discerns which path serves the ultimate goal. Whether you choose wisely matters less than recognizing the choice exists at all—because manipulation doesn't force your hand, it blinds you to the fact that you *have* a hand to play.

If you don't take control of your mind, someone else will. Advertisers will. Social media algorithms will. Your worst habits will. The martial artist trains the mind to make decisions subconsciously that will produce the best outcomes. Putting self-respect into action—choosing long-term excellence over short-term comfort. Not many people make millions of dollars by accident, it requires careful cultivation to bring consistent success. Others are attempting to mentally program you right now, so you must train your mind to avoid scripts written by those that would exploit your energy, and intentionally train it for the outcomes you want.

Your training partners aren't just people to spar with—they're part of your mental armor. Spending quality time with friends, family, and your martial arts community releases oxytocin, the hormone that binds mothers and children, partners and teammates. Research shows oxytocin lessens the sensation of pain and fear, which is why martial artists who train in strong communities often maintain greater courage and pain tolerance than solo practitioners. Choose your community wisely. Surround yourself with people who hold you accountable to your internal locus of control.

Training The Mind

Mental sharpness isn't a permanent state—it's a constantly maintained condition, like a blade that requires regular honing. Here are specific methods that develop the cognitive abilities we've discussed. These aren't random drills—each targets specific neural pathways that enhance combat performance.

Practical Exercises to Sharpen focus

Theory without practice is philosophy. Practice without theory is chaos. Your brain is a muscle. It adapts to the demands you place on it. If you only train your brain to scroll social media and binge streaming content, that's the brain you'll bring to a fight. If you train it to process multiple inputs simultaneously, excellent hand–eye coordination, high threshold of pain tolerance, and to maintain focus through chaos, that's the weapon you'll deploy when it matters.

Each drill targets specific neural pathways that enhance combat performance. Dual–task training develops your ability to think strategically while executing techniques. Spatial exercises sharpen your awareness and distance judgment. Memory challenges strengthen pattern recognition and instant recall. Neurobic tasks build comfort operating without your dominant senses, preparing you for the disorientation of real conflict.

The key is consistent practice. Five minutes daily produces more results than an hour once a week. These exercises feel awkward at first—that's the point. Discomfort means your brain is adapting, building new connections, expanding capacity. Start with the exercises that feel most challenging. That's where you need the most growth. Here's what actually works:

Dual-Task Exercises (Divided Attention Training):

- Hit a bag while reciting the alphabet backwards
- Shadow box while reciting a poem or doing mental math
- Practice techniques while counting backwards from 100 by sevens

These exercises force your brain to process physical and cognitive tasks simultaneously, mimicking the mental demands of actual combat where you must think strategically while executing techniques.

Memory Challenges: Practice techniques in sequences, then reproduce them from memory. This strengthens pattern recognition and recall under pressure. Start with three-move combinations, then five, then ten. The goal is instant recall without conscious thought.

Enhanced Spatial Training:

- Navigate familiar spaces with eyes closed (safely!)
- Estimate distances before measuring them
- Practice catching objects in your peripheral vision
- Mirror exercises where you copy someone's movements exactly

Neurobic Tasks (Dr. Lawrence Katz):

- Eat with your eyes closed (enhances non-visual sensory awareness)

- Punch a bag with your eyes closed (develops proprioception and feel)
- Shower with your eyes closed (builds comfort without visual reliance)
- Count starting at first and last to center and back: 1, 10, 2, 9, 3, 8, 4, 7, 5, 6, then reverse: 5, 6, 4, 7, 8, 3, 9, 2, 10, 1 (cognitive flexibility)
- Breathe in meditation with double count: 1 inhale 1 exhale, 2 inhale 2 exhale, 3 inhale 3 exhale. Make the count in your head with conviction (combines breath control with focused attention)

NOTE; *Proprioception is the body's sense of its own position, movement, and orientation in space, allowing for coordinated movement without conscious thought.*

Kata is Visualization

Kata (Japanese for "form") is a choreographed sequence of movements that simulates combat against imaginary opponents. In Karate, Tae Kwon Do, Kung Fu, and many traditional martial arts, kata represents the collective wisdom of masters who refined these patterns over generations.

Why do martial artists spend years perfecting kata when they could just spar more? Because kata solves a fundamental training problem: **How do you practice techniques at full speed and power without a partner and without injury?**

Sparring teaches timing, distance, and adaptation against a resisting opponent. But in sparring, you hold back. You can't throw full-power strikes to your training partner's throat or practice techniques designed to break joints. Kata lets you practice these techniques at maximum intensity without harming anyone.

But kata's real power lies in neuroplasticity—how it rewires your brain. Repetition builds neural pathways. The first time you perform a technique, your brain creates a weak connection. Do it ten times, and the path becomes clearer. A thousand times, it's a road. Ten thousand times? It's a superhighway.

Each focused repetition strengthens the neural pathways associated with those movements. The technique becomes more deeply embedded. Your body learns not just the individual motion but the transitions between motions, the breathing patterns, the weight shifts, the state associated with proper execution.

Masters practice the same kata for decades because they're not just playing a broken record over and over—they're deepening the neurological grooves that make those techniques automatic. When you need a technique in combat, you don't have time to think through the steps. The thousands of kata repetitions have already programmed your nervous system to execute without conscious thought.

In a real confrontation, your conscious mind processing speed is roughly 200–300 milliseconds. Your trained automatic response through kata repetition? About 100 milliseconds. That split-second difference means your block is already complete while your conscious mind is still recognizing the incoming punch.

Kata bridges the gap between knowing and owning. It's the difference between "I learned this technique" and "this technique is now part of my nervous system." When performed with intent—visualizing opponents, executing with full commitment, breathing correctly—kata creates the same neural activation as actual combat.

Traditional martial arts have always emphasized forms heavily, because they understood neuroplasticity before neuroscience existed. They knew that the fighter who practices forms for an hour daily will execute techniques automatically.

Application In Combat

Every serious practitioner has touched it at least once. Maybe in sparring, maybe in competition, maybe in a moment of genuine danger where everything suddenly became very simple and very clear. You weren't thinking. You weren't performing. You were just — there. Completely there. Moving without deciding to move. Responding before your conscious mind had finished forming the question.

That was your nervous system operating the way it was always designed to — without the interference of the most disruptive element in the equation.

You.

Sport psychologists call it peak performance state. The Zen tradition has called it flow for centuries. The terminology doesn't matter. What matters is that you recognize what it feels like — because if you can recognize it, you can stop accidentally breaking it when it arrives.

It feels like this.

Fear disappears. Not suppressed — genuinely absent. The internal commentary goes quiet. The part of your brain that normally runs a constant background monologue of *what if, am I good enough, what does this look like* — simply stops broadcasting. Time does something strange. A thirty-second exchange feels like it lasted long enough to make considered decisions inside every moment. Sound becomes selective. The crowd, the corner, the noise — all of it falls away. What remains is only what matters. Your opponent. The space between you. The next half-second.

Your body is doing everything without asking permission. The autonomic nervous system — breathing, heart rate, reflexes, the motor patterns drilled so deep your muscles memorized them — running clean, without conscious thought in the way.

Conscious thought, for all its utility, is slow. It analyzes. It second-guesses. It narrates. In a fight, narration is a liability.

The fighter who is thinking *I should throw the jab here* will always be behind the fighter whose jab has already left before the thought fully formed.

Flow state is what training is actually building toward. Not just fitness. Not just technique. The gradual transfer of capability from the thinking mind to the body itself — until the body can be trusted to act while the mind stays clear and present and out of its own way.

You cannot manufacture this state on demand. Anyone who tells you otherwise is selling something.

What you can do is build the conditions that make it likely.

Train until your techniques stop being decisions. This takes longer than most people are willing to invest, which is exactly why most people never get there. A technique you have to think about is a technique your opponent has time to answer. You want movement so deeply grooved that thinking about it would only slow it down.

Walk into every conflict — in the ring, in the boardroom, anywhere — with a clear objective and nothing else. Scattered intention produces scattered performance. Know what you're there to do. Commit to it. Let everything else fall away.

Stay in the present moment with a ferocity that borders on obsessive. The outcome is not your concern while the fight is happening. The next exchange is your concern. The next breath. Flow state cannot survive a mind that has already traveled to the scorecards.

Trust your training the way you trust your balance when you walk down stairs — completely, without verification, without a conscious checklist. The moment you start auditing your own movements mid-execution you have already left the state.

The first time you access it fully you will understand immediately why people dedicate their lives to this pursuit. Not for the trophies. Not for the recognition.

For this.

For the rare and extraordinary experience of being completely alive in a single moment, with every system firing in concert, without fear, without doubt, without the noise that fills most of a human life.

The more familiar it becomes, the shorter the distance to get back there. That is what the years of training quietly build toward — not just a better fighter.

A cleaner mind.

Out-thinking Your Opponent: The Mind as Primary Weapon

Sun Tzu wrote: "The supreme art of war is to subdue the enemy without fighting." When conflict arises, two systems compete for control: your primitive limbic system (fight-or-flight, pure reaction) and your prefrontal cortex (strategic thinking, pattern recognition, risk assessment). The warrior trains to keep higher brain function online when everyone else defaults to primal response.

Your opponent is operating on emotion—anger, ego, fear masked as aggression. Their limbic system has hijacked their decision-making. They're predictable. They're committed to a single path. They've already lost strategic flexibility. You, with a trained mind, are running calculations they can't access: environmental factors, legal implications, social dynamics, exit strategies, threat assessment, de-escalation pathways. You're playing chess while they're throwing rocks.

Operating in cognitive dominance. You are functioning at a higher level because you're processing information faster and more comprehensively than they can. Your training has built neural pathways that allow you to recognize patterns, assess genuine threat level, and identify multiple response options —all while maintaining emotional control. They have one option: escalate. You have ten.

The Mental Skill of De-Escalation

Mental acuity under stress is the mark of a fully developed warrior. When a situation develops—that pre-fight buildup, the tension before commitment—your brain enters its most valuable operational mode. While their amygdala floods them with cortisol and adrenaline, narrowing their focus to pure aggression, your trained prefrontal cortex stays online, processing:

- Threat authenticity: Is this person actually dangerous or performing aggression to mask fear?
- Social dynamics: Who's watching? What's their relationship to the conflict? Can they be leveraged for de-escalation?
- Environmental factors: Exit routes, barriers, witnesses, legal implications
- Opponent psychology: What does this person need to save face and walk away?
- Cost-benefit analysis: What's the actual risk versus the ego-driven impulse to engage?

A great warrior can talk all the way to the edge of physical altercation—not because they're afraid to fight, but because their brain is sophisticated enough to recognize that most conflicts have better solutions than violence. Probing, testing, assessing, buying time for higher cognition to find the *optimal path*. You're engaging their frontal lobe through conversation, giving them space to access their own higher thinking instead of staying locked in reactive aggression. This is literally allowing cooler heads to prevail – you are encouraging them to leave the raw emotion state and actually think.

A calm voice, steady posture, and coherent communication do something powerful: they model regulated behavior. Mirror neurons in their brain start mimicking your state. You're literally using your nervous system to influence theirs. You are deploying advanced mental warfare—using neurobiology to shift them from limbic rage to frontal lobe reasoning.

Why This Matters Legally and Practically

If the situation proceeds to violence despite your efforts, witnesses confirm your attempts at resolution. It is more than just legal strategy—it's proof that your higher brain stayed engaged while theirs didn't. You maintained executive function. You assessed alternatives. You offered exits. They refused every cognitive off-ramp you provided.

But more importantly: you always win if you don't fight. Not because fighting is scary—you've trained for that. Because unnecessary conflict is a *failure of intelligence*. Every fight you avoid through strategic thinking is energy conserved, legal risk eliminated, injury prevented, and reputation enhanced. The opponent who forces you to fight has revealed their mental limitations. The warrior who resolves conflict without violence has demonstrated cognitive superiority.

Being calm and intellectually engaged during confrontation isn't natural—it's trained. Your limbic system wants to react. Your ego wants to dominate. Your trained prefrontal cortex overrides both, calculating the smartest move in real-time. This is what separating the developed mind from the untrained one looks like under pressure.

Some confrontations require verbal push, even controlled aggression in tone, to establish boundaries. We aren't running counter to the warrior ethos—it's using every tool available. But even aggressive communication can serve de-escalation if delivered with strategic intent rather than emotional reaction. You're still thinking. They're still reacting. That gap (the pause) is everything.

The first rule is simple: you always win if you do not fight. Fighting should be reserved for circumstances where your higher brain—after processing all variables—determines it is the best and only option, that no other option exists. Looking for fights or having a low threshold for engagement means your limbic system is still in charge. The sharp mind seeks challenges but avoids unnecessary conflict, because intelligence recognizes the difference between proving yourself and protecting yourself.

This mental skill—maintaining cognitive function under stress, out-thinking the opponent, finding optimal solutions in real-time—is what this entire chapter has been building toward. All the intelligence, wisdom, knowledge, and training converge in the moment someone tries to drag you into their primitive brain state, and you read the trap. You stay sharp. You get strategic. You win with your mind.

Remaining calm and coherent with slick intellectual banter that de-escalates a conflict is a skill of great value and one I continue to struggle to master—hence the writing of this book, to get all my thoughts out so that I can reflect on them in the physical realm. Teaching to learn.

Ultimate Goal

> "You are the living library. You have access to everything already. All you need to do is go inside yourself to find the information you need." Matthew Black. 2018

It's an enigma wrapped in metaphor. Your brain stores every experience, every lesson, every technique you've ever trained. The challenge isn't storage—it's retrieval. The information is there. The question is whether you've organized it in a way that allows rapid access when needed.

The Living Library

Think of it like this: A library with books randomly scattered is useless. A library with a cataloging system is powerful. Your mind is the same. Training creates the cataloging system. Repetition creates the neural pathways that let you access stored information quickly.

When you train a technique a thousand times, you're not just building muscle memory—you're creating an indexed entry in your neural library that can be recalled instantly. When you study strategy, you're building mental models that let you recognize patterns and retrieve relevant responses.

The "going inside" part means trusting your training. In the moment of action, you don't have time to consciously search through everything you know. You need to have trained so thoroughly that the right response emerges automatically from your internal library. It explains what the old masters meant by "mind like water"—calm surface, but vast depth accessible instantly when needed.

Your training is building this library. Every session adds volumes. Every technique creates new cross-references. The more you train, the more comprehensive your internal library becomes, and the faster you can access what you need when you need it.

Mushin: No-Mind

In Japanese martial arts, there's a concept called "mushin"—no-mindedness. It's the state where action happens without conscious thought, where your training responds faster than your thinking can process.

No-mindedness differs from single-mindedness, where you focus intensely on one goal or technique. Single-mindedness is how you train. No-mindedness is how you fight.

Single-mindedness during training: "I will perfect this combination. I will drill it a thousand times. I will break down every element until my body knows it without thinking."

No-mindedness during combat: Your opponent throws a punch. You don't think "block, counter, step." Your body is already moving. The block is already there. The counter is already landing. Thought would slow you down.

The ultimate goal of training in martial arts—to sharpen

your mind so thoroughly through deliberate practice that when the moment arrives, you can get out of the way and let your trained body execute.

Your conscious mind is powerful for planning, analyzing, and strategizing. But in the chaos of combat, conscious thought is too slow. You need to have done the thinking already—during training, during visualization, during thousands of repetitions—so that when action is required, your response is automatic.

We train the mind not to think faster in the moment, but to have already thought so completely that thinking becomes unnecessary.

You now have the foundation for mental mastery—intelligence developed through training, wisdom acquired through experience, knowledge applied strategically, and the state of no-mind where action flows without thought.

Guard your thoughts. What you allow into your mind determines what comes out in your actions. Feed your mind with knowledge, challenge it with complexity, sharpen it with focused training. The fight is won or lost in your head long before fists fly.

A dull blade can't cut. A dull mind can't win. Sharpen both daily.

CHAPTER 11 – SPIRITUAL ACTIVATION

"We all have inner demons to fight. We call these demons 'fear' and 'hatred' and 'anger'. If you do not conquer them, then a life of a hundred years is a tragedy. If you do, a life of a single day can be a triumph."—Yip Man, 1966

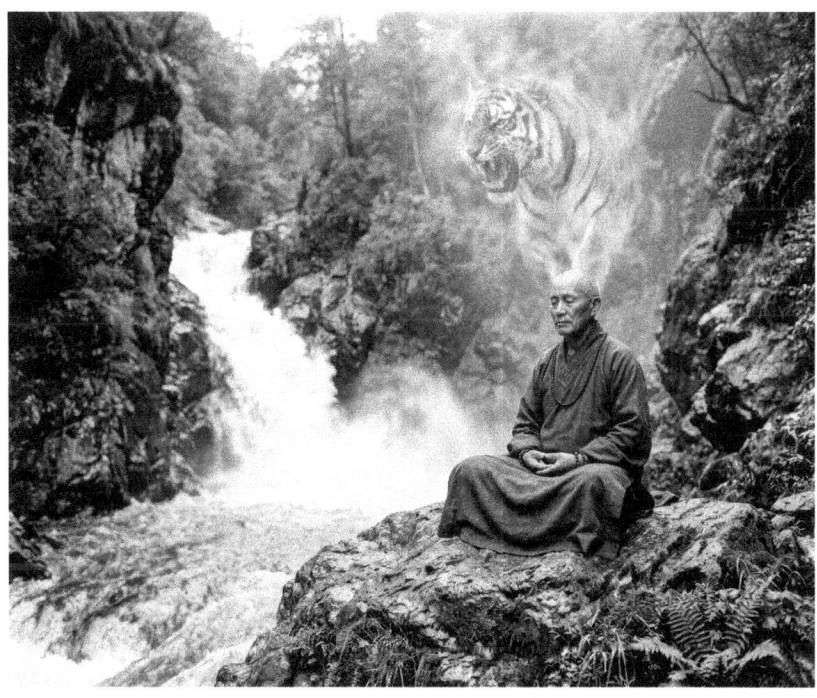

Conquer Your Inner Demons

These are the real opponents. Physical opponents are just the manifestation. If you conquer your inner demons, a single day can be a triumph. If you don't, a hundred years is a tragedy.

Spiritual activation is how you conquer those demons. Not by suppressing them. Not by denying them. By transcending them through presence, through connection to your higher self, through the practices that make you spiritually unshakable.

Fight Beyond the Physical

You've trained your body. You've sharpened your mind. These two dimensions – physical and mental – are what most fighters train. They're enough to make you competent, maybe even good. But there's a third dimension that separates good fighters from unstoppable ones: a force that operates beyond muscle and beyond thought: spiritual activation.

The past is a story we tell ourselves—unreliable, distorted by emotion and time. The future is a phantom that hasn't arrived and may never come. There is only now—this breath, this heartbeat, this moment as you read these words. When you finish this sentence, it will already be memory. If your mind wanders and you think about tomorrow, you've already left reality.

Every moment that passes transforms into memory—subjective, unreliable, reshaped by how we felt rather than what actually happened. The past carries the weight of regret and heartache. The future breeds worry and anxiety. Both are thieves, stealing your attention from the only territory you can actually control: right now. Worry is like sitting in a rocking chair—it feels like you're doing something, but you're getting nowhere. Remind yourself, worry will not add one hour to your life, but will steal momentum. Do not worry. Plan, prepare, meditate—but leave worry behind. It wastes time and energy.

If you're not fully present in the reality you're experiencing, you miss everything that matters. You lose the ability to respond, to adapt, to survive. Your opponent's shoulder drops a fraction before the strike—but you're replaying yesterday's defeat. Your training partner's guard opens for half a second—but you're obsessing over next week's test. The information was there. You just weren't.

The spiritually activated warrior exists in the now. When you release the grip of past regrets and future anxieties, you free your mind to perceive what's actually happening in front of you. An unclouded awareness sees the truth of the moment, not the distortions of fear or wishful thinking.

Living and being present allows you to be focused and aware of what is. Feeling the energy and the applying of all your senses to your surroundings and everything in it. This sensitivity is a vital tool for the master of Martial Arts.

Winning Before the Fight Begins

Battles are often won before they even begin. This happens through mental and spiritual intimidation—shows of force and skill that break an opponent's will before the first strike lands.

Pre-fight, opponents size each other up. They display their best techniques in public warm-up drills. Speed and prowess deftly executed can demoralize other participants. It may seem like just showing off— but it's actually spiritual warfare. You're projecting confidence, capability, and an aura that says: "You don't want this fight."

A spiritually activated warrior controls this realm. They understand the metaphysical battlefield is where the fight is actually decided.

Reading the Soul of Your Opponent

Imagine you were able to read into the soul of an opponent and know exactly how much fight they had in them, and what it would take to make them quit and give up. A spiritually in-tune warrior can sense this, and with practice and polish, they can win without fighting because they know how to posture and make the opponent waver in their resolve.

It isn't operating on prayer or futile wish thinking. It's an observable reality in every combat sport and street encounter.

What You're Actually Reading

The idea of reading someone's soul sounds mystical until you understand what's actually happening. What experienced fighters perceive isn't supernatural — it's a high-resolution scan of micro-signals that most untrained observers filter out entirely.

The hesitation before commitment. Every attack requires a decision, and that decision creates a micro-pause — a fraction of a second where the body is loading before it launches. Beginners miss it. Experienced practitioners have seen it thousands of times and their nervous system flags it before their conscious mind has processed what it saw.

Eye tracking reveals intent in ways people rarely control. Where someone looks before they move tells you where they intend to move. Eyes that avoid yours signal anxiety or deception. Eyes locked too hard, signal overcompensation — someone performing confidence they don't fully possess.

Breath is perhaps the most reliable signal of all because almost nobody manages it consciously under pressure. A fighter whose breathing has gone shallow and rapid is running on adrenaline and depleting fast. One who exhales fully and breathes from the belly is still operating within themselves. You can hear this. You can sometimes feel it in the clinch before you can hear it.

Body language operates below the level of deliberate control. Doubt shows up in the shoulders before it shows up in the feet. Overconfidence shows up in the chin, in the dropped guard, in the slightly wider stance of someone who thinks they've already won. Jerky, disconnected movement signals that the body and mind aren't communicating cleanly — that technique is being consciously assembled rather than fluidly executed. Smooth movement means the opposite: the person you're facing has done this enough times that their body is running ahead of their thinking.

Taken individually, any one of these signals could be misread. Read together, across the first few seconds of an exchange, they produce something that feels to the experienced fighter like intuition — a felt sense of who they're dealing with and what's coming. That feeling isn't mystical. It's pattern recognition operating faster than language. Thousands of hours of standing opposite real opponents has built a database the conscious mind can't access directly but the nervous system consults constantly.

The gap between a fighter who has this and one who doesn't is significant and largely invisible from the outside. Both fighters can throw the same punch. Only one of them already knows it's coming.

How This Manifests in Combat

A fighter enters the ring radiating confidence. You feel it immediately—not bravado, it's genuine belief. Their spiritual warrior is activated. You adjust your strategy accordingly.

Another opponent comes in tentative, despite their skills. You sense the doubt. You apply pressure not just physically but spiritually—through sustained eye contact, through unwavering forward movement, through the energy you project. Their will cracks before their body fails.

Champions often say they "knew" they would win before the fight started. They read their opponent's spiritual state and recognized victory was already decided. The physical fight was just confirmation.

Soul and the Second Self

We exist in a realm much bigger than the physical world we touch and taste every day. Humans across all cultures and all time have held a nearly universal belief: we possess a soul, an unseen aspect operating in parallel with our physical existence.

I believe this soul is an indestructible component that can be rallied to work in tandem with your body, giving you an edge in challenges. Awakening the strength of your soul manifests as an indomitable inner spirit—a deeply ingrained, fierce determination that can be called upon in times of great challenge.

With a disciplined mind, a honed body, and a vigilant spirit working in harmony, you can converge on demand the total innate energy we all possess and direct it toward the challenge you're facing.

I have heard fighters describe being able to summon a powerful force inside themselves that feels supernatural. They talk about tapping into a dimension where time moves slower, where they can act and react much faster, thinking at super speed while moving in a smooth, calm flow state.

Make it a goal to be able to marshal up all of who you are and project the sum of your second self into a single point in time. I assure you that you can train to be able do it, and when you do execute it, in that moment, nothing will be able to stop you.

Understanding Your Second Self

Think of it this way: Your body has limitations. It gets tired. It feels pain. It can be intimidated. Your physical mind can doubt, can overthink, can freeze under pressure.

Your second self—your spiritual warrior—has none of these limitations. It's the part of you that emerges in moments of crisis when you do things you didn't think possible. It's what mothers tap into when they lift cars off their children. It's what soldiers access when they push through wounds that should have stopped them. It's what fighters find in the fifth round when their body is screaming to quit but they somehow continue.

You've probably felt glimpses of it:

– The sparring session where you were exhausted but somehow found another gear

– The moment you got hit hard but your body kept fighting automatically

– The competition where time seemed to slow and you saw everything clearly

– The street encounter where fear should have frozen you but you moved with calm precision

That's your second self. Most people only access it accidentally in moments of extreme need. The spiritually activated warrior learns to summon it on demand.

How to Activate Your Second Self

1. Recognize it exists.— Stop thinking of yourself as one entity with fixed limitations. You have reserves you haven't accessed.

2. Practice summoning it in training.— When you hit the wall in conditioning, when your body says stop—that's when you practice calling on your spiritual warrior. Push past the quit signal. Find what's beyond exhaustion.

3. Use breath and intention.— Before intense training or competition, consciously invite your second self forward. "I call on my spiritual warrior. I activate my full capacity. Physical and spiritual, working as one."

4. Visualize the merger.— See your physical self and your spiritual self overlapping, becoming stronger together than either could be alone.

5. Trust it in combat.— When pressure comes, when fear rises, when your body wants to retreat—trust that your second self is there. It won't let you quit. It won't let you fail. It's indomitable.

We aren't operating in delusion or activating self-hypnosis. It's accessing the deepest reserves of human capability that evolution built into us for survival. You're not creating something that doesn't exist—you're activating what's always been there.

Flow State in Combat

Sport psychologists call this "the zone." Fighters call it different things—being "locked in," having "it," or just "knowing." Zen refers to it being in "the flow." Whatever you call it, it's a real, measurable state where:

- Your perception of time changes—you see strikes coming in slow motion
- Self-consciousness disappears—no internal dialogue, just action
- Performance feels effortless—techniques execute automatically
- Confidence is absolute—you know what to do before thinking it
- Pain and fatigue register but don't affect you

Meet your second self fully activated. Your body and spiritual warrior operating in perfect synchronization.

How to Cultivate Flow

Flow isn't random luck. It has conditions:

Challenge-Skill Balance: You're most likely to enter flow when the challenge slightly exceeds your skill level. Too easy and you're bored. Too hard and you're anxious. Right at the edge—that's where flow lives.

Clear Goals: You know exactly what you're trying to achieve. In sparring: land the combination. In competition: execute the game plan. Clarity invites flow.

Immediate Feedback: Combat provides this naturally. Every technique either works or doesn't. Every movement gets immediate results. This tight feedback loop supports flow.

Complete Focus: No distractions. No phone. No crowd. Just you and the challenge, and why meditation practice is crucial —it trains the focused attention that flow requires.

You can practice entering flow:

- During intense bag work, focus solely on rhythm and power
- In kata, perform with absolute commitment and visualization
- In technical drilling, seek the state where techniques flow without conscious thought
- In conditioning work, push past the quit point and find the calm beyond exhaustion

The more you visit flow in training, the more accessible it becomes in combat. Your spiritual warrior learns the path and can guide you there when needed.

In classical martial arts, this force is sometimes equated with chi, qi, or ki energy. But I believe those terms refer to the greater universal life force that flows through all things. What I'm referring to is something more personal—a second version of you that exists whether you recognize it or not.

You've found your energy. Your spiritual warrior. The part of you that doesn't tire, doesn't fear, doesn't quit. It exists in parallel with your physical self, and when you activate it, you become more than the sum of your parts.

Adapt Without Breaking

Bruce Lee taught: "Be like water." It's become cliché, but the principle is ruthlessly practical. Water doesn't fight containers—it fills them. It doesn't resist obstacles—it flows around them. It can nurture or destroy, soften or erode, depending on what's required. It adapts without losing its essential nature.

In combat, this means rigid fighters break when their game plan fails. The spiritually flexible fighter adapts continuously: opponent circles left, you cut angles and trap them. They switch stances, you adjust entries. They check your leg kicks, you go upstairs. They pressure, you give ground and counter. They retreat, you flow forward. You note they always step directly backward from your front kick—you devise a combo to exploit it.

A spiritual flexibility: adaptability combined with inner indifference to the changes required. No emotion. Simple acceptance. Water doesn't argue with the riverbank. It accepts what is and flows within it. Your spiritual warrior operates the same way—total commitment to the objective, *zero attachment to the method*.

Beyond the Mat

This principle extends far beyond fighting. When life throws a setback, don't crash against it and break. Flow around it. Find another path. When your training partner is bigger and stronger, don't match force for force. Redirect their energy. When emotions threaten to overwhelm you, don't fight or deny them. Let them move through you, then return to your essential calm.

The rigid break. The flexible endure. The spiritually activated warrior understands this deeply. They don't force their will against immovable objects. They find the path of least resistance to maximum effect—not weakness, but tactical intelligence.

Training Spiritual Flexibility

Develop multiple responses to the same attack. Practice transitioning smoothly between ranges. Get comfortable in every position—standing, clinch, ground. Train yourself to see opportunities where others see problems.

In sparring, never commit to one strategy. Always have contingencies. When something doesn't work, abandon it instantly and flow to the next option. Practice against different styles, sizes, skill levels. Learn to match or deliberately mismatch energy.

In life, hold your values firmly but your methods lightly. When your plan fails, adapt without emotional resistance. When circumstances change, change with them. Remember: flexibility is strength. Rigidity is the precursor to breaking.

Water is the most powerful force in nature not because it's hardest, but because it's unrelenting. It adjusts, redirects, finds another way. Nothing can ultimately resist it. Your spiritual warrior operates the same way—relentless adaptation until the objective is achieved.

Training Water-Like Adaptability

Adaptability isn't a personality trait — it's a trained capacity, and like every trained capacity it degrades without deliberate practice and sharpens with it. Here's how you build it across the three domains where it matters most.

In technique, the work is building multiple responses to the same problem. Most practitioners drill one answer to each attack, which means one answer is all they have when pressure comes and the primary option closes. Train at least two or three entries, counters, and transitions for every common situation you face. Practice moving between ranges — striking to clinch to ground and back — until the transitions stop feeling like gear changes and start feeling like one continuous motion. Develop real comfort in every position, not just the positions your style favors. Comfort is the precondition for opportunity. Discomfort narrows attention to survival and blocks everything else out.

In sparring, the discipline is refusing to marry a single strategy. Walk in with a game plan and adjust it the moment the evidence says it isn't working. Have a second option ready before the first one fails, and a third behind that. When a technique stops working against a specific opponent, abandon it immediately — not after two more attempts, immediately — and find what the situation is actually offering. Seek out training partners who challenge your defaults: people bigger and smaller than you, grapplers if you're a striker, strikers if you grapple, practitioners of styles you don't recognize. Each one forces your system to solve a problem it hasn't pre-loaded an answer for. That process of solving unfamiliar problems under pressure is exactly what adaptability is made of.

In life, the same mechanics apply with different variables. When a plan fails, the first and most important response is the absence of emotional resistance — not because the emotion is wrong, but because resistance to what has already happened is energy spent on something that cannot be changed. Adapt to what is, not what you planned for. The values that guide your direction stay fixed. The methods you use to move in that direction stay flexible. Rigidity in method is how capable people get broken by circumstances that would merely redirect someone operating with more give in the system.

Water is instructive not because it's poetic but because it's mechanically accurate. Water never abandons its nature and it never stops moving toward its destination. It simply refuses to exhaust itself fighting obstacles that can be gone around. The river doesn't mourn the rock. It finds the line of least resistance and continues. Nothing ultimately stops it because it never commits to a path that stops it — it commits only to the direction.

Two fighters of identical physical skill, identical technique, identical conditioning — what separates them is the interior. The one who can manage their perceptions, regulate their emotional state under pressure, and access something beyond the purely physical has a genuine advantage that no amount of additional physical training can close. Fighters at the highest level consistently report this — and coaches at the highest level consistently observe it.

The Western world has largely dismissed our ancestors' spiritual wisdom as ancient religious dogma—outdated and overblown. This is a mistake. Spiritual strength, like strength, requires cultivation. Whether through supportive community, spiritual convictions, or disciplined practice, the warrior who develops their spiritual dimension gains access to reserves of strength that pure physicality cannot provide. The Western tendency to dismiss interior development — spiritual practice, emotional regulation, the cultivation of something beyond the measurable — as soft or superstitious has produced technically excellent fighters who come apart under specific kinds of pressure. The traditions that produced the most durable warriors across history, without exception, invested as seriously in the interior development of their fighters as in the physical. Not as religion. As training. As the deliberate cultivation of reserves that purely physical preparation cannot reach. *The warrior who builds only the body has built half a weapon.* The warrior who builds body, mind, and the interior dimension has built something that holds together under conditions that break everything else.

Guard Your Spiritual Energy

Focus on what is beneficial and helpful. Positive energy will make you glow with vitality. Guard your thoughts and what you allow into your mind. Do not dwell on negative concepts or ideas that will lead you to addictions and mental weakness. What we think, we become.

Learn to listen to your inner voice—your spiritual guidance

system. This voice knows truth when your conscious mind is confused. If something feels wrong, it is wrong, and you will live to regret ignoring that feeling.

Listen carefully anytime you hear that internal alarm that says what you're doing is wrong. Stop. Turn around immediately. It will be too late if you don't. Your conscience is your spiritual compass. Follow it.

Throughout history, warriors have understood the spiritual dimension of combat. Militaries employ chaplains to strengthen soldiers' spiritual conviction—to assure them they fight on the side of God and what is righteous. Is this a manipulation? Maybe. But it's recognition that spiritual certainty enhances physical courage.

Some researchers have explored whether human intention affects physical reality. Masaru Emoto's water crystal experiments, while controversial and not accepted by mainstream science, suggested that water exposed to positive intentions formed more symmetrical crystals than water exposed to negative intentions. Whether or not the experiments prove what Emoto claimed, the underlying principle resonates with warriors across cultures: your intentions matter.

Similarly, the famous double-slit experiment in quantum physics demonstrates that observation affects outcomes at the subatomic level. While this doesn't mean "thoughts create reality" in the magical sense, it does suggest that consciousness and physical reality interact in ways we're only beginning to understand.

Here's what matters for the warrior: regardless of the mechanism, countless fighters across centuries have reported that their mental and spiritual state directly affects their performance. Intention matters. Focus matters. Belief matters.

You don't need to understand quantum physics to know that when you enter a fight believing you'll lose, you probably will. When you enter believing in your training, your spirit, and your purpose, you access reserves you didn't know you had, and will probably win.

Feelings are a part of your spiritual existence. Learn to reach out and read a room. Understand the vibe. This is the sixth sense that martial arts masters possess—the ability to know the intentions of others and predict danger before it manifests.

Not some supernatural garbage. It's hyper-awareness trained to the point of instinct. You walk into a bar and immediately sense tension. You meet someone and know instantly they're dangerous. You feel eyes on you before you see who's watching. It can be felt in your gut, when goosebumps pop up on your skin, and the hairs on your neck and arms standing up, often before you even consciously register a threat. Masters have cultivated this skill and they use it everyday.

What the Masters Are Sensing

Nobody tells you this part when you start training. They teach you the techniques, the combinations, the positional theory. All of it useful. None of it the whole story.

The whole story starts much earlier than first contact.

Walk into a room and within seconds you've already assessed it — who's relaxed, who's agitated, who's performing confidence they don't actually possess, who's the most dangerous person present. You didn't run a checklist. You didn't consciously analyze anything. You just knew. Most people dismiss that knowing as vague social instinct and move on.

Martial artists learn to read it like a language.

Watch someone's breathing before they move. Not the big obvious breath that telegraphs a committed attack — the subtle shift that happens in the seconds before. The chest that tightens slightly. The exhale that doesn't quite complete. The rhythm that changes when the decision has been made but the body hasn't moved yet. The decision always arrives in the breath before it arrives in the limbs.

Watch the weight. Before any significant movement the body must shift its center of gravity — imperceptibly, briefly, but definitely. A beginner plants and commits. An experienced fighter gives nothing. But even the most disciplined body cannot defy physics entirely. The tell is always there. The question is whether you've trained your perception fine enough to catch something that exists for a fraction of a second.

The jaw. The hands. The shoulders. These are where tension parks itself when someone is preparing violence. The jaw tightens. The hands make micro-adjustments toward closed. The shoulders move in ways that are neither relaxed nor fully committed — caught between states. Deception lives in the face. Intention lives in the body. Read the body.

And then there is the thing that is harder to explain and easier to dismiss and which every experienced fighter knows is absolutely real.

The Japanese call it sakki. Killing intent. The quality of presence that someone carries when they genuinely mean to harm you — as distinct from someone sparring, someone posturing, someone performing aggression for an audience. It registers before any observable signal. Before the posture shift, before the breathing change, before anything your rational mind could point to and say — there, that's why.

Gavin de Becker wrote about this extensively in the context of civilian self-defense. The body's threat detection system is ancient — older than language, older than conscious reasoning, built during an era when reading another creature's intent was the difference between surviving the encounter and not. It did not disappear when we built cities. It went quiet under layers of social conditioning that taught us to override it in the name of politeness.

The veteran fighter stops overriding it. They stop explaining away the feeling that something is wrong because nothing is technically wrong yet. They act on the signal before the situation provides the evidence — because by the time the evidence arrives, the window for intelligent response has often already closed.

This is why mat time cannot be fully replaced by anything else. You can study this in a book — including this one — and understand it intellectually without developing the capacity at all. The capacity comes from thousands of hours of standing opposite real human beings who are genuinely trying to hit you, throw you, submit you. Hours of your nervous system cataloging signals, building pattern recognition so deep it stops being thought and becomes instinct.

A master isn't processing more data than a beginner. They stopped processing and started perceiving. The distinction matters more than it sounds. Processing is conscious, sequential, slow — the beginner sees a movement and runs it through analysis before responding. Perceiving is pattern recognition operating below the threshold of conscious thought — the master's body is already answering before the mind has filed a report. What masters teach their senior students is how to accelerate that transition, working through four stages of expanding awareness.

The first is environmental. Every room you enter contains information you're not collecting if you walk in looking at your phone or your destination. Before you look directly at anything, scan the space. Exits, structural features, positioning of people relative to each other and to you. Who arrived before you and where did they place themselves. The emotional temperature of the room — whether the energy is relaxed, cautious, wound tight, or artificially calm in the way that precedes something. This sounds like paranoia until you practice it long enough to realize it's simply attention redirected. Most people move through environments almost entirely blind to them. The first stage of awareness training is just learning to look.

The second stage narrows from the room to the individual. One person at a time, building a real-time read from the signals they're broadcasting without knowing it. Body language, breathing, the quality of attention they're giving their surroundings. Practice predicting what someone is about to do before they do it — in conversation, in traffic, in sparring. In training, work specifically on sensing your partner's intention before the movement begins. The setup always precedes the strike. The weight shifts before the feet move. The decision registers in the body before the body executes. Learning to read that preparation gap is the beginning of operating ahead of events rather than behind them.

The third stage moves into territory that makes some people uncomfortable because it operates below the level of what can be cleanly articulated. Intuitive sensing — the felt knowledge that something is wrong before anything observable confirms it. The hair on the arms. The tightening in the gut. The sudden sharpening of attention without an identified cause. These aren't superstition. They're your threat detection system filing a report through channels older than language, channels that bypass the conscious mind because conscious processing is too slow for what they're designed to handle. Meditation develops this capacity not by making you spiritual but by quieting the cognitive noise that drowns these signals out in most people. The discipline is learning to distinguish genuine danger awareness — which has a specific physical signature — from general anxiety, which is a different sensation entirely once you've trained yourself to notice the difference.

The fourth stage is projection. Having developed the capacity to read intent in others, you learn to manage what you project. A calm, grounded, genuinely capable presence communicates something to people around you that most cannot name but all register. People who intend harm are reading their environment constantly, assessing targets and resistance. Someone who moves with quiet certainty, whose attention is full and unhurried, who occupies their space without apology or aggression — that person rarely gets selected. The projection of false intent is the advanced application: the ability to appear open when you're closed, passive when you're loaded, unaware when you're completely aware. Masters use this in combat as freely as they use technique. The warrior's deepest paradox lives here — the person most capable of violence is often the one least required to use it, because what they carry is readable to anyone paying attention, and most people, when they read it clearly, recalculate.

Martial Arts Training for Sixth Sense

Traditional kata teaches this. You visualize opponents attacking from different directions. You practice sensing their intent before you see them, training your subconscious to process threat signals.

Randori (free practice against multiple attackers) develops it further. You can't watch everyone, so you learn to feel the attack coming. Your peripheral awareness expands. Your intuition sharpens.

The best training? Experience. Every sparring session. Every competition. Every situation where you had to read someone quickly. Your sixth sense is like a muscle—use it or lose it.

Sixth sense develops through:
– Consistent presence and awareness training
– Meditation that sharpens your receptive capacity
– Experience reading body language, micro-expressions, energy
– Trusting your gut instead of rationalizing away what you feel

The spiritually activated warrior doesn't dismiss these feelings as imagination. They honor them as information often life-saving data.

Foundation: Connecting Body and Spirit

All of these spiritual practices—presence, reading energy, connecting with your second self—require a foundation: deep connection with your body. You can't activate your spiritual warrior if you're disconnected from the vessel it inhabits. We build this connection methodically, starting with breath, progressing to meditation, and culminating in the Matt-Meditation-Method (MMM). Each builds on the last. Each prepares you for the next. Let's break them down.

Advanced Breath Work

Breath is the bridge between body and spirit. Master your breath, and you master your state.

The Technique:

1. **Inhale** — Slow, deep breathing through your nose. You can alternate nostrils by gently closing one side at a time if you wish. Extend your belly and use your diaphragm to pull in maximum oxygen. Fill your lungs completely, then pull in that extra bit your diaphragm can give you.
2. **Hold** — Slow count to 5.
3. **Exhale** — Think the word "RELAX" as you breathe out through pursed lips, slowly. At the end, when no more breath can be expelled, use three or four movements of your diaphragm to push out the final bit of air remaining.
4. **Hold** — No air in the lungs. Slow count to 5.
5. **Repeat** — 10 complete cycles.

This breath work oxygenates your blood, calms your nervous system, and centers your energy. Practice it daily. Use it before training, before competition, before any moment where you need to access your full capacity—physical and spiritual.

Breath is life. Control your breath, control your life force.

Meditation: Cultivating Presence

In Chapter 7 we have covered meditation techniques, but lets expand on the concept of meditation which has been employed for millennia as a tool for spiritual activation. At its core, meditation is being present and listening intently. Prayer, by comparison, is talking and asking. One is reception, the other transmission. The warrior needs both, but meditation—the art of receptive awareness—is what activates your spiritual senses. But you can use this tool in motion and not just sitting still in lotus position. Meditation in action forms your sixth sense.

Use it while operating and fully functional, being completely present but seeing the world spiritually. Don't just try to see your surroundings. Feel them. Sense the energy in a room before you enter. Notice the shift in atmosphere when tension rises. This sixth sense develops from being aware of all things around you and in your path. It is possible to meditate while doing activities, try this while gardening, or walking in nature and meditate on your internal being, while remaining open to the energy around you. Sense what is, perceive what the eye cannot see. This is how to become sensitive enough to have "eyes in the back of your head."

This meditation while in the present—this living fully in the now—opens the doorway to your deeper power. Once you've established breath control and meditative awareness, you're ready for the final practice that unites all three dimensions.

The Matt-Meditation-Method: Body Dialogue and Self-Love

Now we combine stretch, breath, and meditation with conscious intention. The Matt-Meditation-Method (MMM)—a practice that creates meaningful connection between your physical self and your spirit. Engaging in the highest state of spiritual activation that will help develop your sixth sense with a heightened mind/body connection. There is energy all around us, we just need to connect to it in meditation.

MMM Practice:

Find a calm environment. Close your eyes and see a white screen with nothing on it, feel the electrical energy flowing through your body. When you are ready open your eyes and prepare to stretch for at least fifteen minutes. You'll move slowly and patiently, giving conscious attention and love to each different body part.

  I. **Select a body part** — Start at your feet. Hold them physically with your hands.
  II. **Make contact** — Touch this area. Make a comprehensive connection. Acknowledge it consciously to confirm your positive intention.
  III. **Express gratitude** — Tell that spot you recognize it. That you appreciate it. That you cherish it. These aren't just thoughts—speak them internally with conviction.
  IV. **Breathe and stretch** — Inhale deeply through your nose and hold. As you hold, elongate into a deeper stretch. Continue the positive attention to your chosen body part. Exhale slowly through your mouth.
  V. **Hold the position** — Maintain each stretch for around one minute, staying present with that body part the entire time.
  VI. **Progress systematically** — Work your way up: feet, ankles, calves, knees, thighs, hips, core, back, shoulders, arms, neck, face. Each area gets a few moments of attention, gratitude, and love.

Active dialogue occurs while stretching. You're not just moving through positions—you're having a conversation with your body, acknowledging every part that makes your life as a warrior possible.

Example in Practice:

Stretch into a sitting split and hold each ankle. As you hold them, tell them you love them. They are the only two ankles you will ever have. Stretch your back and talk to your organs. Appreciate them. Stretch your shoulders—did you know spiritualists claim we carry our sadness in our left shoulder? Show your left shoulder, and your right shoulder, some love. Tell them you appreciate the work they do for you every day. Having problems with your teeth? Take a few calm minutes to thank them for their tireless, on-demand work they've done thus far. Nutrition is important for health, and so is self love.

Adaptation For Injuries

If you have a particular injury or area you want healed find the best position to be in to touch that area. Start with a peaceful mind and move your being into a state of gratitude. Being thankful for your wonderful self healing systems, all the little pieces of you that come together to make you healthy. Touch and caress the injured area (or as close as possible) and give thanks for it and ask it to accept the healing blood flow and visualize your life force, your bio electrical energy moving to the injury and warming it up. Ask and feel energy moving inside of you and from both inside and from your touch sense the subtle movement of the energy to the target area. Do this for 15 minutes each day until fully recovered.

Why This Works

Don't confuse this with feel-good nonsense. There's real science here, and there's warrior logic ingrained.

Neurological Benefits:

- Increased body awareness enhances proprioception (knowing where your body is in space)
- Focused attention on specific areas increases neural con-

nections to those regions
- Mind–body integration improves, leading to better movement control

Psychological Benefits:
- Self-compassion reduces performance anxiety
- Body appreciation increases motivation to train and protect what you value
- Positive self-talk rewires negative thought patterns

Physical Benefits:
- Conscious stretching with intention improves flexibility beyond passive stretching alone
- Attention to specific areas can reduce chronic pain and tension
- Grateful awareness increases mindful training, which means fewer injuries

The Warrior Logic:

Think about this: What happens when someone attacks someone you love? You go the extra mile to defend them. You find strength you didn't know you had. You become fierce.

If you loved yourself more—if you truly loved and appreciated your body—imagine how that translates when it comes time to defend yourself. I'm not promoting narcissism or ego stroking. I'm recognizing that your body is your partner in this journey. It deserves your respect, your care, your love.

The Core Principle:

Your body and all its parts get ignored too often. We only recognize a body part when it hurts. We complain and sometimes curse our aching back or sore shoulder. But when was the last time you thanked your body for what it does right?

Stop. Stretch. Touch and hold your body. Understand it is the only one you will get. Love it—because what's your other choice? To abuse and hate it? To ignore it? No.

Fighters who practice the Matt–Meditation–Method report faster recovery from training, reduced chronic aches and pains, better body awareness during technique work, increased motivation to maintain conditioning, and stronger mental resilience during tough training.

Most importantly, they report feeling more complete—like they're not just training a body, but partnering with it.

You will get health and healing when you send love and recognition to your body's soldiers on your physical front line. A spiritual activation through body connection.

Practice all three: advanced breath work to control your state, meditation to cultivate presence, and the Matt–Meditation–Method to connect body and spirit. Together, they form the foundation upon which your spiritual warrior stands.

Summation of Spiritual Activation

We have discussed the need to live fully present, in reading the energy and intention of those around you before they've consciously committed to action. We've explored your second self—the spiritual warrior who doesn't tire, doesn't fear, doesn't quit—and begun the practice of letting this part of you surface when needed. Through breath work and the Matt–Meditation–Method, you've established dialogue with your own body, learning to listen to what it tells you and respond with the care it deserves. You've cultivated the state where time stretches, awareness sharpens, and action flows without thought. You've trained yourself to be like water—flexible enough to adapt, powerful enough to overcome, patient enough to find the path of least resistance to maximum effect.

These aren't separate skills. They're facets of the same diamond—your complete self, awakened.

The warrior who trains only the body becomes strong but brittle. The warrior who sharpens mind and body but neglects spirit remains incomplete, like a blade with no handle—dangerous but difficult to wield. When all three dimensions align —body honed, mind sharpened, spirit awakened—you become something greater than the sum of your parts. You step onto the mat and your opponent feels it before you move. They can't name what they're sensing, but somewhere deep in their soul, they recognize they're facing someone operating at a different frequency.

Spiritual activation manifests in practice like a warrior with an extra sense to navigate with. Almost supernatural. You, fully present, fully integrated, fully capable of accessing everything you've trained. Your body executing with precision. Your mind processing without interference. Your spiritual warrior standing beside you, calm and relentless, guiding you through chaos with the certainty of someone who's already seen the outcome.

The fight you're preparing for—whether on the mat, in the street, or navigating the conflicts life throws at you—doesn't start with the first punch. It starts in the spiritual realm, where presence confronts absence, where calm meets chaos, where the activated warrior recognizes the path before the untrained even see the obstacle.

You have the tools. You know the practices. Now comes the only part that matters: doing the work daily. Five minutes of breath work before training. Fifteen minutes of body dialogue after. Moments of full presence throughout your day. The spiritual warrior isn't built in a weekend seminar—it's forged through consistent practice, the same way yourself was built through thousands of reps and your consciousness was sharpened through years of study.

Complete yourself. Not someday. Not when you have more time. Not after you've mastered everything else. Now. Today. This moment. Because the spiritually activated warrior understands something the rest don't: there is only now, and now is when the work happens.

Step onto your path as the complete warrior—integrated and self aligned. The world needs fewer half-formed fighters and more integrated human beings who've done the hard work of becoming whole.

Access your sixth sense. Activate your spirit.

CHAPTER 12 – FLOW IN ZEN

"The way of the sword and the way of zen have the same purpose, that of killing the ego."—Yamada Jirokichi, 1965

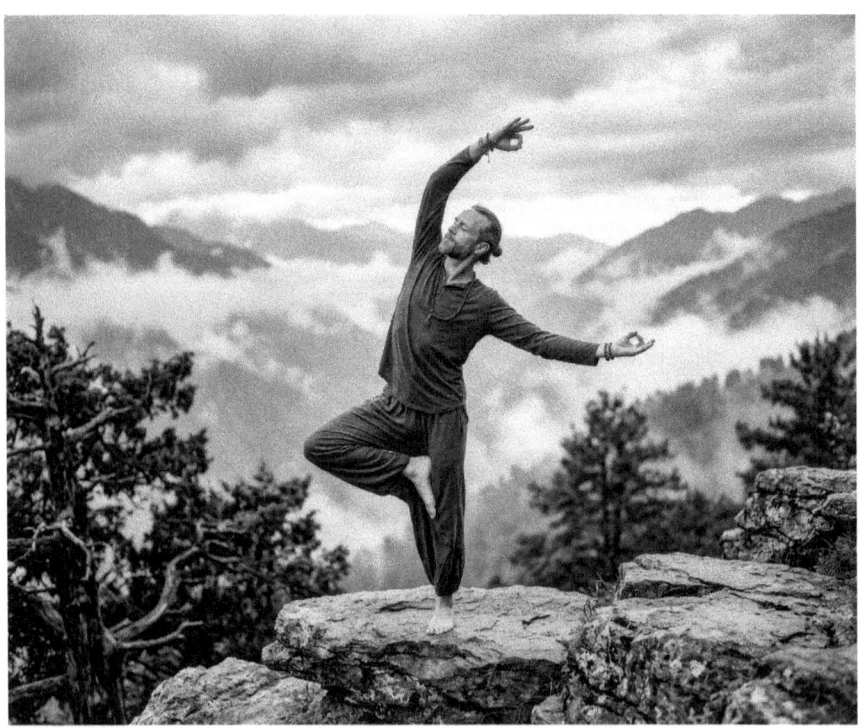

What is Zen

You've felt it—everything slows down, your body moves without instruction, your opponent telegraphs every move. You're not thinking, you're being. In that moment, you're unstoppable because fear and doubt don't exist—only action exists.

This is Zen. This is flow. This is what you've been training for since your first day on the mat.

Most fighters chase this state but never understand it. They experience it randomly, lose it immediately, and spend years trying to find it again. They don't realize that flow isn't something that happens to you—it's something you cultivate. It's a skill, like any other. And like any skill, it can be trained.

This chapter will show you how to find that state, live in that state, and fight from that state. Not occasionally. Consistently.

Defining Zen for Warriors

Many have heard of Zen but few can describe it. Fewer still live it. Here's why: Zen can't be intellectualized. You can't think your way into Zen—that's the opposite of Zen. You have to experience it, then learn to recognize it, then train to access it on demand.

Let me give you the clearest definition specific to warriors that I can distill:

Zen is the state where your conscious mind gets out of the way and lets your trained self execute.

That's it. Strip away the cultural trappings and religious packaging, and Zen is simply this: being completely present in the moment, perceiving clearly, acting without hesitation, and doing so from a state of mental stillness rather than mental noise. Zen equals no-mindedness.

Why This Matters

Remember learning your first combination? Jab–cross–hook. Your conscious mind had to direct every movement: "Okay, jab with the left. Now twist and throw the right. Okay, now bring the hook—wait, which hand?"

Slow. Clunky. Ineffective. Your mind blocks everything else out. Picture being in intense real combat with total focus only on your movements—you're dead.

Now, after a thousand repetitions, someone says "jab–cross–hook" and your body just does it. Smooth. Fast. No thought required. The conscious brain is free to process separate information while your body moves automatically.

That's the beginning of Zen. Now imagine experiencing that with everything—every technique, every defensive reaction, every tactical adjustment. Your body knows what to do before your mind realizes what's happening.

Three Stages of Mastery

Stage 1: Conscious Incompetence — You don't know what you're doing. Every movement requires deliberate thought. You're awkward, slow, constantly correcting. Everyone starts here.

Stage 2: Conscious Competence — You can execute techniques correctly, but only when you think about them. You're functional but not fluid. Speed and pressure expose your limitations. Most martial artists plateau here.

Stage 3: Unconscious Competence (Zen) — Your body executes without conscious direction. Techniques flow automatically. You respond faster than thought allows. This is Zen in combat.

You reach Stage 3 through *mindful repetition* followed by *mindless execution*. You train consciously—paying attention to every detail, correcting every flaw, ingraining every movement deeply. Then, in the moment of action, you release conscious control and trust what you've built.

The Line Between Mind and Spirit

Here's an exercise that changed my understanding of my existential being.

Sit quietly. Close your eyes. Empty your mind as much as possible. Just breathe. Just exist.

Eventually, a thought will appear. "I'm hungry." "My knee hurts." "I wonder if I locked the door."

When that thought appears, ask yourself: *Who* is thinking this thought? And more importantly: *Who* is observing the thought?

If you're observing your thoughts, who's doing the thinking? You are not your thoughts. You're the one *watching* your thoughts. Which means there's a you beneath the you that you think you are. Your body is one layer. Your mind is another. Your thoughts are another. But there's something deeper still—something observing it all. The realm of person–hood—of existence itself—is so much bigger and deeper than I ever imagined.

My conclusion? There is a spiritual dimension where the real you resides, meaning, you're not just a body moving through space. You're not just a mind solving problems. You're something far more profound—**a consciousness experiencing itself, layer by layer, discovering depths you didn't know existed.** This took some time for me to understand, so lets see where it takes us next, and if need be, you can mark this spot for further review. I suspect it to be a very individual and personal enlightenment that needs to be experienced, not just explained.

At this juncture we are now straddling the border between mind and spirit, but where is that and why does it matter? Let's get simplistic and boil it down to the core elements. Your mind generates thoughts. Your spirit—your deeper self—observes them. In Zen, you learn to operate from the observer, not the thinker.

An unconditioned mind generates thoughts during combat: "He's bigger than me." "I'm getting tired." "What if I lose?" These thoughts slow you down. They create hesitation. They inject fear and doubt into what should be pure action.

Your spirit—trained well—doesn't generate these thoughts. It simply responds. It sees the opening and moves. It feels the threat and counters. No commentary. No judgment. Just action.

Learning to fight from your spirit instead is what separates good fighters from great ones. The mind analyzes. The spirit acts.

Marks of Zen

As you develop Zen, two qualities become evident to everyone around you:

Disciplined — Every morning, you face a choice: train or don't train. Work or don't work. Improve or stay the same. Discipline is perseverance against your base desire for comfort. It's choosing the hard path when the easy path is right there, available, tempting. When you choose to work hard and better your life repeatedly, relentlessly, discipline becomes your identity. Not something you do. Something you *are*.

Composed — I've watched students lose composure in their first sparring sessions—hit and panic, emotions running uncontrolled, technique abandoned, flailing. Then months later, those same students are calm under fire, centered under pressure, focused on their goals even when chaos surrounds them. Composure is being unfazed in the face of fear and uncertainty. It's maintaining control of your state when everything around you screams "lose control." Say this to yourself every day: "I am in control." Mean it. Believe it. Become it.

Train For Zen

Attaining Zen isn't mysticism. It's trained deliberately through specific practices that rewire how you process combat.

Method 1: Observe Your Thoughts

Daily, for five minutes, practice observing your thoughts without engaging them. When a thought appears, notice it: "There's a thought about being hungry." Don't analyze it. Don't follow it. Just observe and return to breath.

This trains you to recognize the difference between the thought-generator (mind) and the thought-observer (spirit). In combat, this becomes the difference between "I'm thinking about defending" and simply defending.

Method 2: Override the Quit Signal

During hard training—when you're exhausted and your mind screams to quit—pause for just a moment. Notice the thoughts: "I can't do this." "I need to stop."

Recognize those are thoughts, not truth. Then choose to continue anyway. You're training your spirit to override your mind's survival instinct.

Method 3: Kill the Commentary

When sparring, catch yourself narrating your experience internally. "He's fast." "I'm doing well." "That hurt." Every time you notice internal commentary, deliberately release it, push it out and make your mind clean. Return to pure perception and action.

Over time, the commentary quiets. What remains is pure flow—your spirit moving your body in response to what is, not what your mind thinks about what is.

Method 4: Overflow Drilling

Pick one technique or combination. Drill it until you can't anymore. Then drill it fifty more times. Push past the point where your conscious mind checks out from boredom. That's when your unconscious mind takes over and the technique becomes truly automatic.

Most people stop training when they can perform a technique correctly. Masters train until they can't perform it incorrectly.

Method 5: Sensory Deprivation Practice

Train with your eyes closed. Remove one sense and force your other awareness systems to compensate. Shadowbox in darkness. Hit the bag blindfolded. Drill techniques without visual feedback.

This forces you out of visual-cognitive processing and into pure kinesthetic awareness—feeling the technique instead of seeing it. This is closer to the Zen state.

Method 6: Rhythm Training

Bruce Lee was the 1958 Crown Colony Cha-cha champion of Hong Kong. He spoke of fights having a certain rhythm or beat, and the ability to break or flow with that rhythm was a key component of his Jeet Kune Do philosophy.

Train to music with a strong beat. Let the rhythm carry your movement. Don't think about timing—feel it. Your techniques synchronize with the rhythm automatically. Then train in silence. Notice how the internal rhythm remains. That's your body learning to generate flow without external cues.

Additional Tools:

Develop a pre-performance ritual—deep breathing, specific stretches, a mental phrase. The key is consistency. Eventually, the ritual itself triggers the Zen state because your brain associates it with flow.

After every session, identify the moments where you felt flow. What preceded them? What state were you in? Track this over weeks and months. Patterns emerge. You learn your personal pathway into Zen.

When I Lost My Zen

Late 2020. COVID hysteria had the world by the throat. The dojo closed, then reopened with restrictions that made real practice impossible. I was working from home, boundaries between work and life dissolved, consuming a constant stream of fear and division without filter, without discipline, without the observer stance I'd spent years cultivating.

I thought I was handling it. I thought I was fine.

I walked into Dr. Manjit Gosel's office for a routine checkup. Dr. Gosel holds a second-degree black belt in Shotokan. We'd worked together for years—our appointments usually involved as much discussion about martial arts and combat strategy as bloodwork and supplements.

He took one look at me and said, "You've lost your Zen."

We'd never explicitly talked about Zen. Not once. Yet he saw it immediately. Or rather, he saw its absence.

"What?" I said, more defensively than I intended.

"Your Zen," he repeated, calm but certain. "You don't have it anymore. I can see it. You're tense. You're carrying everything in your shoulders. Your breathing is shallow. You're not centered.

He was right. I'd been feeling off from all the fear and hype pushed through the media and I hadn't meditated on it. The world and the future felt uncertain. The confidence I usually carried had been replaced by a continuous hum of low-grade anxiety I couldn't shake. The peace I'd cultivated had evaporated, replaced by agitation I tried to ignore.

I'd let external chaos become internal chaos, and I hadn't even noticed the transition. I wasn't self-examining.

I'd abandoned the check-in process and meditation practice when I needed it most. I'd let the observer fall asleep and the thinker take over completely—analyzing threats, processing news, catastrophizing futures that never did happen.

I went home that day and sat in my training room for an hour. Just breathing. Just observing thoughts without following them. Just existing in the present moment without judgment.

It took weeks to fully recover what I'd lost. Weeks of daily meditation, drilling basics with complete focus, deliberately releasing the tension and anxiety I'd been carrying.

But it came back. Slowly, then suddenly. One day I was working the Mook Jong (wooden dummy) and felt it—the old flow, the familiar calm, the observer watching the mind while the body executed without interference. Everything clicked again, but it had taken 3 months.

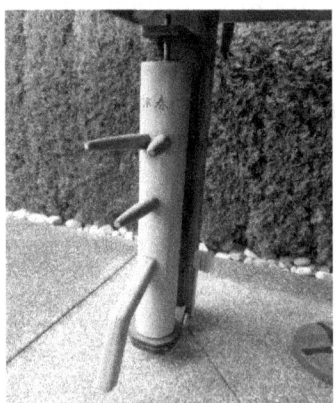

Here's what I learned: **Zen isn't a permanent achievement.** It's a state you maintain through practice. Stop practicing, and it fades. The longer you go without it, the more you forget what it feels like, and the easier it becomes to accept its absence as normal.

When you notice the signs—and you will—you know what to do. The training methods aren't just for building Zen. They're for recovering it when life knocks you off center. Because life will knock you off center. Count on it.

What Zen Feels Like

You're sparring. An opening appears. You don't think "jab-cross-hook." Your body is already throwing the combination before your conscious mind registers the opportunity.

You're exhausted, gassed, ready to quit. But your body keeps moving. Techniques keep flowing. You find reserves you didn't know existed.

You're facing a bigger, stronger opponent. Logically, you should be scared. But you're calm. Centered. You see their tells. You time your counters. You flow like water around their strength.

That's Zen.

What Zen Feels Like

You're sparring. An opening appears. You don't think "jab-cross-hook." Your body is already throwing the combination before your conscious mind registers the opportunity.

You're exhausted, gassed, ready to quit. But your body keeps moving. Techniques keep flowing. You find reserves you didn't know existed.

You're facing a bigger, stronger opponent. Logically, you should be scared. But you're calm. Centered. You see their tells. You time your counters. You flow like water around their strength.

That's Zen.

Knowing Where You Are

Some sessions you walk out and can't fully account for what happened in there. Not because it went badly. Because it went somewhere beyond your normal operating range and the usual vocabulary doesn't quite cover it. You moved well. Better than well. Things worked that you didn't consciously decide to do. Time behaved strangely. The noise of the gym receded to somewhere that wasn't your concern.

You know the feeling. The question worth asking is whether you understand it well enough to notice when it's present — and catch it early when it's gone.

Inside that state the most obvious sign is what's missing. The running internal monologue — the part that scores your performance in real time, that winces at mistakes and congratulates itself on clean exchanges — simply isn't there. Not quieted. Absent. Your techniques stop arriving as decisions and start arriving as facts. Your opponent moves and your body has already begun answering before the observation has finished registering. The fatigue in your legs exists the way weather outside a window exists — acknowledged, irrelevant.

Fear doesn't vanish. Anyone claiming otherwise is either lying or hasn't faced anything genuinely threatening. What changes is its jurisdiction. It's present but it lost the vote somewhere in the middle rounds and it knows it.

When it leaves, it doesn't announce itself.

The first sign is usually a technique that requires assembling. Something that was automatic yesterday now has visible seams — you can feel yourself selecting it, loading it, executing it in sequence rather than as a single unbroken gesture. Then the shoulders climb toward the ears. The jaw takes on cargo it has no business carrying. You're half a beat behind exchanges you were comfortably inside moments ago.

Your training partners read it in your silhouette before you've finished diagnosing it internally. The rhythm is wrong. You're not moving like yourself — and the people who train with you regularly carry a felt sense of what yourself actually looks like that is more accurate than your own assessment in the moment.

The instinct when this happens is to bear down. Dig in. Manufacture through effort what arrived effortlessly before. This is exactly wrong and most people do it anyway because effort is the only tool they trust.

Flow and force don't live on the same street. You cannot work harder into a state that exists precisely where the working stops. The trying is the wall, not the door.

Go back to the breath instead. One real exhale — not a technique, not a reset ritual, just an actual breath that you follow all the way out. Then the next thirty seconds only. Not the round. Not the session. Thirty seconds of honest presence and see what the body remembers on its own.

What accumulates over years of serious training is something that doesn't show up on any record or ranking. A familiarity with this state that gradually reduces the journey back to it. The first time you touched it you probably didn't recognize it until it was already gone. Then you learned to recognize it while it was happening. Then you learned the texture of the moments just before it arrives. Eventually you learn what in your preparation tends to invite it and what in your behavior tends to drive it away.

That is the real curriculum. Running underneath the techniques, the conditioning, the strategy — a slow education in the geography of your own best performance.

The Archer and the Target

In "Zen and the Art of Archery," there's a line that captures the books essence: "The contest consists in the archer aiming at himself—and yet not at himself, in hitting himself, yet not himself, and thus becoming simultaneously the aimer and the aim."

The Zen archery master doesn't calculate distance, wind, angle. He becomes the entire system—the bow, the arrow, the target, the space between. When he releases, it's not him shooting at something separate. It's the universe expressing itself through his trained body.

You're not fighting your opponent. You're fighting yourself.

Every match is against the version of you that wants to quit, that doubts, that fears, that makes excuses. Your opponent is just the mirror showing you who you are in this moment.

When you lose because you gassed in the third round, you didn't lose to your opponent—you lost to your conditioning choices over the past six months. When you lose because fear made you hesitate, you didn't lose to your opponent—you lost to the part of yourself that still needs development.

When you win in Zen, you're not defeating someone else—you're transcending your own limitations.

Application

Before training, focus on becoming the best version of yourself that day. Your training partner shows you where you still have gaps. They're not your enemy—they're your teacher.

During competition, your true fight is internal: Can you stay calm under pressure? Can you execute your game plan? Can you adapt when things don't go as planned?

After every session, ask yourself: What version of me showed up today? The version that makes excuses or faces truth? The version that quits when tired or finds another gear?

Become the System

In Zen, you're not separate from your techniques, your training, your opponent, or the outcome. You're the system. When you fight, you're the entire combat system expressing itself.

This removes ego. This removes fear. What remains is pure function.

The bow doesn't worry if the arrow hits the target. The bow simply does what bows do—release with perfect form. The result follows naturally from correct execution.

You don't need to worry about winning. You simply need to execute with perfect form. The result follows naturally.

That's Zen.

Living in Zen

In Zen, you practice a technique so many times it's forgotten. Then it becomes a permanent tool accessed subconsciously, without thought. Your mind stores the entire program in a file that uploads instantly when needed.

It's when you stop thinking about it that it can be executed perfectly.

This is what all the repetition is for, why masters drill basics for decades. Not to memorize them—to transcend them. To move beyond the clunky think–do, think–do of conscious execution and into the flow of unconscious mastery.

The Zen Path

Everything you do has consequences in a very practical, observable, real-world sense.

You dominate others for personal gain? You create enemies and isolation. You cut corners in training? You get exposed when it matters. You abuse your body? It breaks down. You lie to yourself about your abilities? Reality corrects you violently.

Conversely: You train with integrity? You become capable. You treat people with respect? You build genuine relationships. You face your weaknesses honestly? You transform them into strengths.

This is what Yamada Jirokichi meant when he said the way of the sword and the way of Zen both kill the ego. Not your sense of self—your attachment to image, your need for validation, your fear of being exposed as less than perfect.

When the ego dies, what remains is truth. And truth makes you dangerous.

Ultimate Goal

The ultimate goal of Zen is to realize your complete being—

all that you could be. Not just as a fighter. As a human.

Zen is calm and peaceful, and it's evident to everyone around you. It exudes confidence and clarity. A person in total control, making rational decisions, producing positive outcomes. A quiet fortitude that's impossible to miss.

When you have it, you feel invincible. Not because you can't be beaten—because you don't fear being beaten. You've transcended the ego's need to win and found something deeper: the pure expression of your trained self.

The flow state you're chasing in combat is available in every moment of your life. You can live in flow. You can exist in Zen. A peace through times of stress, fear, shock, pain. A calm, collected confidence that cannot be panicked. An acceptance of reality and real-time circumstances while remaining calmly centered.

Who Are You

To reach Zen requires something most people aren't willing to give: complete honesty with yourself about who you are and who you're becoming.

Look in the mirror. Not at your body—into your soul.

Are you the person you want to be? Are you living with the integrity you claim to value? Are you training with the discipline you preach? Are you showing up as your highest self, or making excuses for why you're not?

Zen isn't a destination. It's a practice. A way of being. A commitment to showing up every day and doing the work even when—especially when—you don't feel like it.

Some days you'll touch flow and feel invincible. Other days you'll struggle with basics that used to come easy. This is the path. Both are necessary. Both are teaching you.

The warrior who only trains when motivated trains occasionally. The warrior who trains regardless of motivation trains consistently. And consistency is what builds mastery.

Your Medicine Is Within

Bruce Lee said it perfectly: "The medicine for my suffering I had within me from the very beginning."

Zen is being in balance with the vessel and all its components. Understanding that all of you needs equal amounts of work and attention. That your mental health needs as much attention and time as you put into your physical self at the gym. Your spirit also requires nourishment and love. All three need work, exercise and nutrition, just in different ways. Understand when one is unhealthy, the whole is sick too. It is a task of refinement and self betterment that continues until your last breath.

An example of the perfect Zen is the balance you feel inside when it all goes right. When you are having the perfect day and all the factors both in your control and out of it, lined up anyway. When you are a little extra calm, content, peaceful, happy. A day when a perfect stranger shows you kindness. When someone you care about is in a great mood too. When the birds seem to sing just for you. When the world smiles and it is all green lights in front of you. That is your Zen moment, and it can be cultivated. It can be more often than just once in a blue moon. When you positively affect yourself, you will affect everything around you too. Yin and yang flowing in harmony.

Meditate on this.

CHAPTER 13 – THE MARTIAL TAO

"The martial way is not picking your fights or picking how things will go, it is adapting to how things are."— Gunnar Nelson. 2017

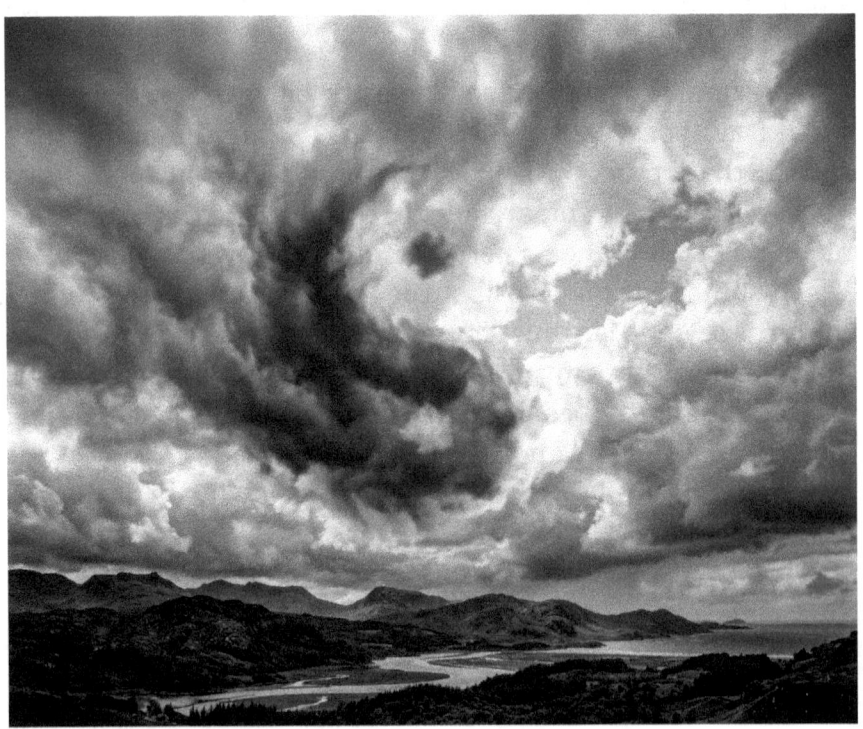

Tao is the small word that expresses an enormous concept. If Zen is the balanced internal flow that moves from within yourself, the Tao is the word for the entirety of external flow as it acts upon you and everything else. Tao means THE ALL, encompassing the universal energy. Enormous concept right?

In the Tao Te Ching, Lao Tzu describes the Tao as representing the ultimate, nameless reality that underlies and unifies all existence—the natural order and flow of the universe that cannot be fully expressed in words or concepts.

The path of living in harmony with the Tao involves embracing simplicity, spontaneity, and humility; accepting the natural cycles of change and transformation; and understanding that opposing forces like yin and yang are complementary rather than contradictory. Rather than imposing one's will on the world, Taoism teaches that true wisdom and effectiveness come from aligning oneself with the Tao's effortless flow.

The Way You Walk Through the World

You've been training for months, maybe years. Your techniques are sharper. Your body is stronger. Your mind is clearer.

But something's still missing.

You can fight, so you are a fighter, *great*—but are you living as a complete and balanced <u>warrior</u>?

There's a difference between a fighter and a warrior. A massive one. Fighting is something you do for minutes at a time. Being a warrior is how you exist *every* moment of *every* day. It's not a skill you practice—it's a path you walk.

The Martial Tao encompasses the balanced way, the warrior's path, the art of living in harmony with reality while being ready for anything reality throws at you.

Most martial artists never make this leap. They train hard, they compete, they even win—but they never truly embody the warrior way. They keep their training in a box labeled "martial arts" and live the rest of their life as civilians.

This chapter will show you how to close that gap. How to take all you've learned—body, mind, spirit—and weave it into the fabric of your daily existence. Not as performance. As identity.

"The Way"?

People ask: What is this "way"? What are its principles? How can you know if you're walking it?

The Martial Tao is living everyday guided by a warriors three responsibilities. Develop yourself and your physicality specifically for conflict. To be proficient and able to adapt to new forms of use to be successful in the arena of life. To develop your mind to foresee, and control the terms of engagement, to be able to avoid any fight not to your mission purpose. Express your indomitable spirit and fight with calm, dignity and total commitment.

The Tao is developing, adapting and expressing all your capabilities for the Martial Arts. That's it. That's the way. Everything else flows from these three.

In addition to war–fighting, Samurai were expected to master an expressive art form like charcoal painting, or haiku. Many became masters of theater as actors, or played stringed instruments and sang. This embrace of opposites, is the reason the Shoguns' warriors, were commanded to spend much of their leisure time practicing soft art forms. A balance of the soul is considered struck if all sides of ones character and capacity are explored from one extreme to the other. In modern application, is this creating an oil painting for every fight we get in? Is it taking a math class for every poetry class? Is it digging ditches for a living but singing opera on the weekends? You decide what it means, but balance of your personality is the goal. A warrior should seek the softer arts to balance the hard arts. Finding the opposite to our strengths to practice and explore is a personal journey, unique for each of us. The perfect Tao is the harmony of your inner duality as one in continual flow with the grand external Tao.

Let me show you what this actually looks like in practice.

Live the Three Responsibilities in daily life, to develop yourself fully and to find ways to excel in all that you do.

Responsibility 1: Develop Your Physicality

Your physicality should be advancing through hard training—that's obvious. But the warrior way means never wasting an opportunity to test and expand your capabilities.

Skip and hop rather than just walk. Take the stairs with gusto, not an elevator. Hike a hill instead of driving around it. Jump across a stream. Climb a cliff. Test all of your physical limits, both big and small.

Why? Because your body is your primary weapon. Every movement is either making it sharper or letting it dull. There's no neutral.

I've watched people transform not through their gym sessions—everyone trains hard at the gym—but through how they moved through their daily life. The guy who sprints to his car in the rain instead of jogging. The woman who carries all the groceries in one trip instead of two. The student who practices balance on curbs while walking to school.

These aren't "workouts." They're expressions of the warrior mindset: I am a physical being, and I will not waste the gift of this body.

Your body is the vehicle for everything else you'll accomplish. Treat it like the irreplaceable instrument it is.

Responsibility 2: Develop Your Mind;

Your mind and body are inexorably attached. If you are doing it right, they should communicate faster and with more precision every day of your life.

Developing your mind isn't just reading martial arts books—though that helps. It's constant mental exercise and physical stimulus woven into daily life. Here are some exercises I use daily;

- Look briefly at a scene, look away and describe, to sharpen your observation and estimation
- Estimate crowd sizes to develop spatial awareness
- Work on hand–eye and foot–eye coordination drills (ie: hand ball, hackey sack)
- Do puzzles quickly to strengthen pattern recognition
- Read tactical situations in everyday environments

The warrior's mind is always working. Always processing. Always preparing.

When you walk into a restaurant, do you automatically scan for exits? Do you position yourself with your back to a solid wall and where you can see the entrances? Do you notice who's paying attention to you and who isn't? Do you notice anomaly's where ever you are? Bulges around waistbands, furtive movements and glances? There is always a lot going on below the surface.

Operating in awareness. It's the warriors mind doing its job: keeping you one step ahead of whatever might come.

Responsibility 3: Develop Your Indomitable Spirit

The indomitable spirit cannot be beaten even when the body has failed. Despite losing, despite facing death, your spirit wills itself to continue to rise, to live and to win.

This spirit inside you—the one that refuses to quit—is honed anytime you choose not to quit when quitting would be easier.

At the gym when your body screams to stop and you do one more rep. On a run when your lungs burn and you maintain pace. In sparring when you're exhausted and you keep your hands up. In life when circumstances crush you and you get up anyway.

Here's the hard truth: the human mind is generally weak. It will beg you to quit long before your body has given 75% of what it's capable of. Your indomitable spirit is the last line of defense against your mind's weakness.

Meditate on this. Your mind will betray you. you will fail you. Your spirit is the only part of you that can't be broken unless you allow it.

So don't.

Yin, Yang & the Tao

Balance isn't staying in the middle—it's flowing between extremes as circumstances demand. This is the Tao: the way of natural harmony through constant adaptation.

The Tao isn't a destination. It's not a state you achieve and then maintain. It's a path—literally, "the way"—that you walk by responding to what is rather than forcing what you want. Water flowing downhill doesn't decide its route in advance. It finds the path of least resistance and follows it, adapting to every obstacle, filling every space, never lost in fighting, instead always moving forward.

The warrior's model for living rejects rigid adherence to plans that become obsolete the moment circumstances change, embracing instead fluid adaptation that maintains purpose while adjusting method. The Tao is universal energy—the force that moves through all things, connecting all of existence. You can fight against it and exhaust yourself, or you can align with it and let it carry you.

The martial artist learns this on the mat first. You can't force a technique on a resisting opponent. You can't muscle your way through superior positioning. But when you feel their energy, their intention, their momentum—and flow with it rather than against it—suddenly impossible techniques become effortless. You're not fighting them anymore. You're redirecting the Tao that flows through both of you.

This principle extends beyond combat. It's the foundation of living as a complete warrior—someone who understands themselves deeply enough to move through life with purpose, adaptability, and power.

Yin and Yang: The Map of Reality

The Yin/Yang symbol encodes this truth in geometry. Two sides flowing into each other, always moving, always whole. One cannot exist without the other. They define each other. They complete each other.

Look closely at the symbol. Within the black, a dot of white. Within the white, a dot of black. Deep wisdom, not just decoration—it's a map of reality, a warning, and an instruction manual all compressed into one image.

Reality, as we experience it, exists through duality. Hot defines cold. Hard requires soft. Advance creates retreat. Victory and defeat. Strength and weakness. Light and shadow. Neither side exists alone; they're locked in an eternal dance, each giving birth to the other, each containing the seed of its opposite.

The white dot in the black warns: even at your strongest, you carry the seed of weakness. Even in your moment of greatest aggression, maintain calm at your core. Even in victory, remember defeat is possible. The black dot in the white reminds: even in peace, hold readiness for war. Even in your most vulnerable moment, strength remains within you. Even in defeat, the seed of your next victory is already planted.

This is the warrior's reality. You are never purely one thing.

You contain multitudes. The question isn't whether you have both light and shadow, strength and weakness, aggression and calm. You do. Everyone does. The question is whether you understand this, accept it, and learn to flow between both sides as circumstances demand.

Most people resist this truth. They want to be only strong, only confident, only victorious. They deny their weaknesses, suppress their fears, hide their vulnerabilities. This creates brittleness. When life exposes what they've been denying, they break.

The warrior who understands yin and yang doesn't break. They bend. They flow. They acknowledge both sides and develop mastery over the full spectrum. This is what makes them complete.

Opposites Attract

To achieve any goal, you must embrace its opposite.

Bravery is built while you are inside fear, not after it's gone. You train while scared — that's the only way the nervous system learns that fear is survivable and that action is possible inside it. Strength requires passing through weakness — the breakdown of muscle tissue under load is the literal mechanism of growth, not a setback on the way to it. Stamina only develops past the point where your body is screaming to stop. Before that threshold you're just maintaining. After it you're building.

Discipline isn't available to the person who already wants to be disciplined. It's built by the person who doesn't want to do the thing and does it anyway, repeatedly, until wanting becomes irrelevant. Respect flows outward before it returns. Peace is found on the far side of chaos, not by avoiding it. Wholeness requires looking directly at what's broken — the person who won't examine their damage stays defined by it.

None of this is paradox for its own sake. It's the mechanical reality of how human development works. Growth happens in the space between opposing states — in the discomfort, the resistance, the moment one condition is pressing against its opposite hard enough that transformation becomes possible. Remove the tension and you remove the growth. The untrained person does exactly that. They avoid fear so courage never develops. They quit when tired so endurance never builds. They optimize for comfort and then wonder why nothing changes.

The warrior seeks this tension deliberately. Not because suffering has value in itself but because the specific capacity you want lives on the other side of the condition you're trying to avoid. You can't transcend what you haven't inhabited. You can't master what you've kept at arm's length.

The yin/yang symbol makes this explicit in its geometry. Within the black, a seed of white. Within the white, a seed of black. The forces don't cancel each other — they define each other, contain each other, require each other. The warrior who has mastered both sides of a duality is more complete than one who has only developed half of it, however impressively. Fierce when the situation demands ferocity. Calm when calm is the more powerful response. Confident without brittleness. Strong without rigidity. The capacity to move fluidly between opposing states — that's not contradiction. That's mastery.

Know Yourself: The Starting Point

General Sun Tzu, writing for the Zhao dynastic armies of ancient China, distilled the warrior's path into one profound statement: "Know yourself and know your enemy, and you have everything you need to win."

Notice the order. Know *yourself* first. Then know your enemy.

It isn't accidental. You can't accurately assess an opponent if you don't first understand your own capabilities, limitations, motivations, and patterns. You can't read another person's energy if you haven't first learned to read your own. You can't flow with the Tao if you're disconnected from your internal state.

Self-knowledge is the foundation upon which everything else builds. Without it, you're fighting blind—not just against opponents, but against yourself.

Here's Sun Tzu's wisdom's applied to the warrior's internal development:

Know your goal — Where are you going? What does the complete version of yourself look like? Not the fantasy version that ignores your nature, but the actualized version that develops your true potential. You can't walk the path if you don't know where it leads.

Know your role — What's your function in achieving it? Are you the leader or the student? The aggressor or the counter-puncher? The scholar, the lover, or the warrior—or all three? Understanding your role means understanding your current position on the path and what's required to move forward.

Know your strengths — What advantages do you bring? Not what you wish you had, but what you actually possess. Physical attributes, capabilities, learned skills, natural talents. The warrior who fights from their strengths multiplies their effectiveness.

Know your weaknesses — What vulnerabilities must you protect? Where do you break under pressure? What patterns sabotage you? What fears control you? The warrior who denies their weaknesses gets exploited. The warrior who acknowledges them can compensate, defend, or—over time— transform them into strengths.

Plan for all outcomes — What if you win? What if you lose? What if something unexpected happens? The warrior who's prepared for every scenario rarely gets blindsided. They might not always win, but they're never unprepared.

This process isn't just for combat. Use it for every significant decision you face. Training. Relationships. Career. Life itself.

But notice: every element of this method of inquiry requires brutal self-honesty. You can't know your strengths if you're inflating your ego. You can't know your weaknesses if you're in denial. You can't know your goal if you're chasing someone else's definition of success. You can't know your role if you're performing a character instead of being yourself.

Self-knowledge demands that you look in the mirror—not at your surface, but into your depths—and see yourself clearly. Who are you really? Not who you present to the world, not who you wish you were, not who your parents wanted you to be. Who are you at your core?

What motivates you? What scares you? What makes you quit? What makes you persist? What do you value above everything else? What would you die for? What would you refuse to die for?

These aren't abstract questions. These are the questions that determine whether you're living your life or performing someone else's. These are the questions that determine whether you can access your full power or whether you're operating at a fraction of your capacity because you're fighting your own nature.

All of creation lives in calculable harmony. Balance exists everywhere—in ecosystems, in geometry, in the waves of resonance frequency that hum the pulse of the Earth. The warrior seeks this same balance, starting with the most important territory they'll ever conquer: themselves.

The Warrior as Artist: Expressing Your True Self

When you achieve this self-knowledge, when you understand both sides of your nature, when you stop fighting who you are and start developing who you are—something shifts.

You stop mechanically performing techniques and start expressing yourself through them.

This is the warrior as artist.

Seeing training through the eyes of an artist makes what you do real, because it personalizes it. It makes everything yours. Sure, someone teaches you and shows you what to do, but now you need to capture it and own it through concentrated effort and repetition.

When you flow as an artist who is expressing rather than just mechanically doing a movement, a strike, a weave, even simply walking—the way you move transforms. Mind and body are brought closer together in disciplined efficiency and artistic interpretation. You're no longer imitating your instructor. You're expressing yourself through the art.

This is what Bruce Lee meant when he said to make the art your own. Not to disrespect tradition, but to filter it through your unique combination of attributes, limitations, personality, and spirit. Two fighters can learn the same technique from the same instructor and express it completely differently—because they're different people with different bodies and different internal landscapes.

The complete warrior understands this. They learn the fundamentals with precision. They drill the basics until they're automatic. But then they find themselves within the structure. They discover how their body naturally wants to move, what techniques align with their spirit, what strategies match their personality.

Nobody is advocating to ignore instruction or invent new techniques from scratch. It's about taking what you've been given and making it yours through the alchemy of self-knowledge combined with disciplined practice.

The martial artist becomes more aware of their surroundings, more alert to potential challenges and challengers in daily interactions. They flow within their environment, feeling energy and attitudes, participating in the experience at a much deeper level than the untrained.

This is what mastery looks like: effortless execution of what was once impossible. The observer sees grace. *You* know it's thousands of hours of deliberate practice combined with deep self-understanding that allows authentic expression rather than mechanical imitation.

When you move through the world this way—grounded in self-knowledge, balanced between opposites, expressing your true nature through disciplined action—you become the living embodiment of the Tao. You're not fighting the current. You are the current.

Assessing Your Balance

Your life is best lived in harmony with your environment. No matter where you find yourself, either your surroundings affect you, or you flow within them. The warrior who understands themselves can maintain their center regardless of external chaos. The warrior who doesn't know themselves gets thrown by every shift in circumstance.

Are you living in balance? Ask yourself this question with brutal honesty: How are you feeling right now?

If you sense irritability, overwhelming anxiousness, trouble focusing, constantly looking for distractions, or avoiding situations—your inner self is trying to communicate. Listen. These aren't weaknesses to suppress. These are signals that something within your system needs attention.

Remember yin and yang. Within your strength, there's a seed of weakness. Within your calm, there's a seed of chaos. These seeds grow when ignored. They shrink when acknowledged.

The 30-Second Check-In

Meditation is the most effective tool for internal communication. Take 30 seconds right now to check in with your internal systems. Get out of the way and let your innate systems talk with each other. Solutions will come to you much faster than if you wait until you hit roadblocks from not paying attention to your well-being.

Is your heart beating hard? Are you frowning, tense, uneasy? Where are you holding tension in your body? What thought keeps circling that you're trying to ignore? What emotion are you suppressing?

Listen and interpret the answers. Do not avoid this work. The cues have become physical and won't go away by burying the feeling. Identifying troubles early ensures your well-being. The warrior who waits until they're broken to address imbalance has waited too long.

You can't always be on a Tibetan mountaintop finding inner peace. But inspiration to look inside can be cultivated anywhere. Find your moments and use them to assess your internal rhythm.

For me, sometimes it was in the flow of motocross racing—inside my helmet, totally engaged in the physically challenging action—when I would suddenly become clear on a nagging feeling. Truth would enter and reveal itself while my mind was engaged in the challenging activity at hand. In the space between the mind being totally occupied, my spirit was free to communicate.

Your moments might be different. Maybe it's during a long run. Maybe it's in the shower. Maybe it's while drilling kata for the thousandth time. The activity doesn't matter. What matters is that you create space for your internal systems to communicate with your conscious mind.

This is the practical application of understanding yin and yang. You're not trying to eliminate the shadow side. You're acknowledging it, listening to it, learning from it. The irritability is telling you something. The anxiety is pointing toward something that needs addressing. The tension in your shoulders is holding something you haven't processed.

The warrior who suppresses these signals becomes rigid. Brittleness follows. Eventually, they break.

The warrior who listens to these signals stays flexible. They adjust. They flow. They address small imbalances before they become catastrophic failures.

The Complete Package

Now we can see how all of this connects to create the warrior living in the Tao—the person who has done the deep work of understanding themselves and can therefore move through life with power, purpose, and adaptability. This power comes from you but also from the Tao. When one with the Tao you are operating with your energy and as a conduit for the universal energy.

You understand duality. You know you contain both strength and weakness, both light and shadow, both the capacity for violence and the capacity for peace. You don't deny either side. You develop mastery over both.

You know yourself. You've done the brutal self-assessment. You know your strengths, your weaknesses, your motivations, your fears, your patterns, your goals. You're not performing a character. You're being yourself—the actual version, not the fantasy version.

You flow with the Tao. You don't fight reality. You don't insist that the world conform to your plans. You adapt to what is while maintaining your purpose. Like water, you find the path, you fill the space, you keep moving forward.

You express yourself as an artist. Your techniques aren't imitations. They're expressions of your unique self filtered through disciplined training. Your life isn't someone else's template. It's your authentic path walked with integrity.

You maintain your balance. You check in with yourself

regularly. You listen to the signals. You address small imbalances before they become big problems. You understand that balance isn't a static state—it's a dynamic flow between extremes.

The complete package. What the Tao demands and what understanding yin and yang enables. What Sun Tzu meant when he said to know yourself first.

You can't be a complete warrior if you don't know who you are. You can't flow with universal energy if you're disconnected from your own. You can't master the external if you haven't mastered the internal.

Everything starts with self-knowledge. Everything builds from understanding your own nature—both sides, light and shadow, strength and weakness, yin and yang.

The warrior's journey begins by looking inward. Here they cultivate their Zen which will lead them to the Tao.

Practical Tao: Maintaining Balance

The Five Pillars

Living in harmony with the Tao requires maintaining five foundational elements: adequate rest, quality nutrition, physical activity, controlled stress, and social connection. These aren't tasks you complete and check off—they're daily commitments woven into how you walk through the world.

1. Seven hours of deep sleep.
2. Food that fuels rather than depletes.
3. Movement that challenges your body.
4. Pressure that builds capacity without breaking you.
5. People who understand and support your path.

Miss any one of these consistently, and your entire system begins to degrade.

The warrior's integrated being operate as one integrated

system. You can't sharpen your mind while running your body into the ground. You can't hone and feeding comprehensively garbage inputs. You can't maintain either while surrounding yourself with people who drain your energy or undermine your purpose. The five pillars work together or they fail together.

Balance Time

Here's the mathematics of your day: seven hours for sleep, three for eating properly, one for meditation and focused exercise, two for travel and transitions. That leaves roughly ten hours for earning a living, personal development, family, friends, community responsibilities, and everything else that demands your attention.

Time is finite. Energy is finite. Every hour spent is energy you can never recover. This creates a forcing function—you must choose what matters because you literally cannot do all that will be requested of you. The warrior who doesn't choose gets their time chosen for them by whomever has the loudest voice, the most urgent demand, or the most persistent request.

Most people organize their days around other people's agendas. They respond to emails, attend meetings that could have been avoided, say yes to requests they should decline, and wonder why they never have time for their own development. Some may confuse it with being generous. It's not, it is abdication.

The solution isn't complex: know what *must be* done versus what *you want* done versus what *others want* done. The first category are the fundamentals that keep your system running. The second category is important but flexible—your personal goals that advance over time. The third category requires brutal filtering—most of what others want from you doesn't actually require your involvement.

Set boundaries. Create space for what matters to you. Learn to recognize when someone is asking for your time because they genuinely need your specific contribution versus when they're asking because you're convenient and you haven't learned to say *no*.

But don't become rigid. Life is unpredictable. The warrior who plans every minute and then falls apart when plans change hasn't achieved discipline—they've created brittleness. Build structure, then practice flexibility within it. Know what's truly non-negotiable versus what's merely your preference. When unexpected situations arise, adapt. The Tao flows around obstacles; so should you.

Tao is Always Present

Living by calendars and schedules creates a trap: you're never actually where you are. You're mentally rehearsing what comes next or analyzing what just happened. Doing so is useful in limited doses—planning prevents chaos, and reflection produces learning. But when it becomes your default state, you've stopped living in the only time that actually exists.

The past no longer exists. It's memory, subjective and incomplete. The future doesn't yet exist. There is only now. The warrior who lives in the past carries regret. The warrior who lives in the future carries anxiety. The warrior who lives now carries only awareness.

In combat, the fighter thinking about the last exchange they lost or the round coming up next is the fighter who gets hit. The fighter who's in the present, reads their opponent in real-time and responds appropriately. The same principle applies outside the ring. The person mentally elsewhere misses information, makes poor decisions, and experiences life through a fog of distraction. Clarity wins over muddled confusion every time. Being in the present (operating within the Tao), manifests that clarity.

The Overthinking Trap

Thinking is necessary. Overthinking is destructive. The

difference is action.

Considering options is wise. Gathering information before deciding is prudent. But endless contemplation without commitment creates paralysis. Worse, it creates a pessimistic mind-frame. While you're mentally cataloging every possible trap and pitfall, you're dwelling on negative outcomes and training your nervous system to expect failure.

The solution is simple but not easy: make a decision. Even an imperfect decision executed with commitment produces information. Overthinking produces only more thinking.

When you catch yourself spiraling—analyzing the same situation for the third, fifth, tenth time without moving forward—interrupt the pattern physically. I use a sharp finger snap and a deliberate breath in through my nose. This signals my entire system that I want full focus, present moment, decision time. Some people tap their fingers in a specific sequence. Others use a physical stance or hand position. The specific trigger doesn't matter. What matters is consistency. Your nervous system learns to associate the physical action with state change.

Train this deliberately. When you notice overthinking beginning, deploy your physical trigger immediately, then commit to a decision within the next sixty seconds. Even if the decision is "I need more information from X source," that's a decision with action attached. Break the loop.

The warrior doesn't need perfect information. They need sufficient information combined with the willingness to act. Perfection is the enemy of progress. You'll never have complete certainty. Move anyway.

Moderation and Self-Correction

When you notice you've been doing too much of one thing—training to the point of injury, working to the point of burnout, socializing to the point of exhaustion, even meditating to the point of disconnection from practical life—examine that pattern. Is it serving your goals or sabotaging them? If it's not, moderate or stop.

This is the Tao in practice. Not rigid adherence to rules, but constant adjustment based on "what is" rather than what you wish. The yin/yang symbol reminds you: within every extreme lies the seed of its opposite. Push too hard in any direction, and you create the conditions for collapse in that area.

Balance isn't a static state you achieve and maintain. It's a dynamic process of constant micro-adjustments. Check in with yourself regularly. Listen to the signals your body and mind send. When something feels off, investigate rather than ignore. Small corrections prevent large failures.

The complete warrior understands this. They maintain the five pillars. They guard their time. They live in the present moment. They think clearly but act decisively. They practice moderation while pursuing excellence. This is how you walk the Tao while living in the modern world—not by retreating to a mountaintop, but by bringing the principles into daily practice through disciplined attention and constant adjustment.

Conscious Tao

The Martial Tao isn't a destination. It's a way of walking through the world.

It's scanning for exits when you enter a room. It's training when you don't feel like it. It's saying no to time burglars. It's checking in with your body before it screams for attention. It's balancing opposites: hard and soft, aggressive and patient, confident and humble.

Most importantly, it's adapting to reality as it is—not as you wish it were.

Gunnar Nelson said it: "The martial way is not picking your fights or picking how things will go, it is adapting to how things are."

That's the Tao. That's the way.

You've learned the three responsibilities: physicality, mind, spirit. You've learned the principle of yin and yang: embrace opposites. You've learned to assess your balance and manage your time. You've learned to live in the present and defeat overthinking.

These aren't separate lessons. They're all pointing toward one fundamental truth.

We Are One Energy

The energy that flows through you is the same energy that flows through your opponent, from the sun, through the trees and their roots reaching into earth. Understanding the Tao—the universal energy that powers all existence, requires a type of unfamiliar humility for the human spirit to strive for. A journey of the soul in the energy fields we are operating in everyday, all around us. A new way of sensing the physical world, through a field of vibrations of a vast life force that encompasses our whole being inside of it.

You and I are made of the same force. We are connected at a level deeper than flesh, deeper than thought, deeper than individuality. When you strike, you're moving universal energy against universal energy. When you breathe, you're exchanging atoms with every living thing that's ever existed. When you train, you're refining your small portion of the infinite whole.

Understanding this changes everything.

Caring for yourself becomes caring for the universal. Caring for your surroundings becomes caring for your own extended body. Harming another without cause becomes self–harm. Cultivating peace within yourself becomes cultivating peace in the world. The distinction between internal and external dissolves.

Have your heard a voice inside that tells you what is right?

Is this the still small voice of God speaking to you? If the Tao is THE ALL and God is energy, then yes. The voice guiding you toward balance, toward growth, toward alignment—that's not separate from you. It's the universal energy recognizing itself through your consciousness.

When you are mentally strong, physically capable, and your spirit flows in harmony with the Tao, the separation between you and everything else becomes transparent. You see through the illusion of isolation. You understand that your daily problems, your fears, your ego–driven conflicts, from the perspective of the infinite, these are ripples on the surface of an ocean so vast it has no shore.

Let's not be nihilistic. Your life matters. Your choices matter. But they matter as part of the whole, not separate from it. The warrior who grasps this, fights injustice not from ego but from recognition: allowing evil to flourish anywhere damages the universal energy we all share. Protecting others becomes protecting yourself because there is no meaningful distinction.

The warrior battles injustice in all its incarnations—not from righteousness, but from understanding. Preventing wrongs, protecting the vulnerable, cultivating peace and balance—these aren't external missions. They're maintenance of the universal energy that flows through everything, including you.

Zen matters because Zen is your individual consciousness aligning with the Tao—the universal consciousness. When you find your Zen flow, you're not creating something new. You're removing the barriers between your small self and your true self, which is inseparable from everything.

You are powered by the Tao. You are nurtured by it. You are made of it. And so is everyone and everything else.

The Hard Road

Now you know the way.

The only question left is: will you adapt and learn to be in flow with the Tao?

Not sometimes. Not when it's convenient. Not when you feel inspired or when conditions are perfect. Daily. In every choice, every movement, every interaction with the universal energy that surrounds and comprises you.

Flowing with the Tao is a narrow path. The road is hard. Few follow it for life.

Be one of the few.

CHAPTER 14 – TEACH TO LEARN

"When you teach someone, both the teacher and the student benefit."—Lao Tzu. 600BCE

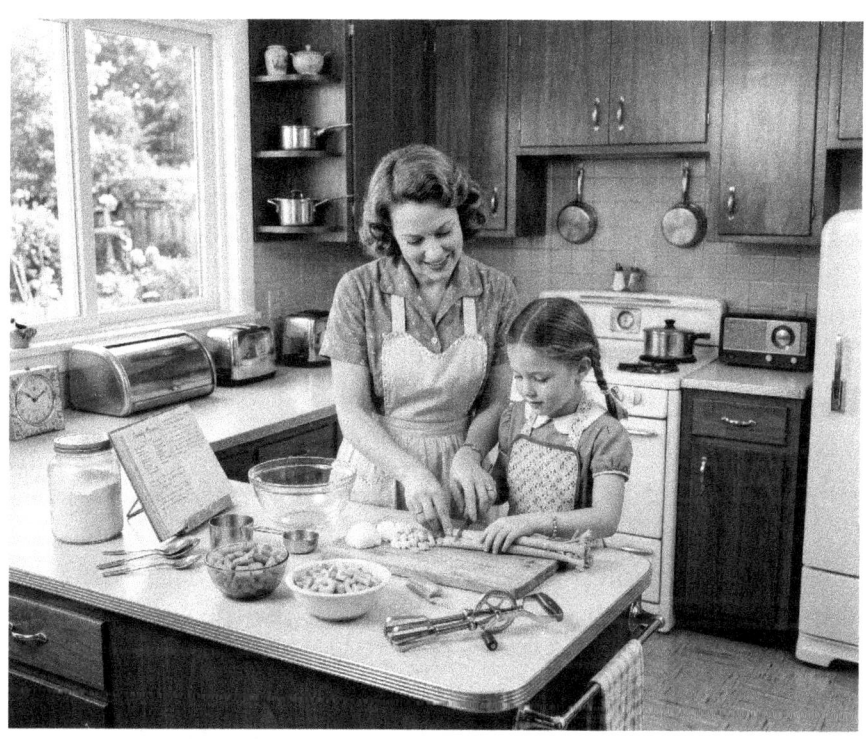

Learning to Teach

You think you know a technique until a white belt asks you 'why' and you realize you've been doing it on autopilot for years.

I was teaching a basic reverse punch—something I'd thrown ten thousand times, something so fundamental I could do it in my sleep. A new student, maybe three weeks in, raised her hand. "Why do we rotate the fist at the end?"

Simple question. I opened my mouth to answer and... nothing. I mean, I knew the answer—I'd been taught it a decade ago, I'd repeated it in forms and drills and sparring—but I'd never actually thought about it. I'd never broken down the mechanics, the physics, the reason. I just knew it worked.

"Uh... it adds power," I said. Which was true, but as useless as a solar powered flashlight. It is an empty descriptor. It was the answer someone gives when they don't actually understand what they're talking about.

She nodded politely, but I could see it in her eyes: that wasn't good enough. And it shouldn't have been. She wasn't asking for a platitude. She was asking for an understanding. And I couldn't give it to her because I didn't have it myself.

That question haunted me for a week. I went back to my instructor. I studied anatomy. I filmed myself throwing the punch in slow motion. I tested it on the heavy bag with rotation, without rotation, early rotation, late rotation. And finally, I understood—not just knew, but understood—how the rotation of the fist aligns the radius and ulna bones in the forearm to create a solid structure on impact, how it engages the lat and creates torque through the shoulder, how the timing of the rotation determines whether you get maximum power transfer or a glancing blow. Some muscles or all the muscles possible recruited to transfer the fastest amount of force.

When I taught the reverse punch the next week, I was teaching something I'd mastered through being forced to explain it. That white belt made me a better martial artist by asking a question I should have asked myself years ago.

This is the paradox of teaching: you think you're the one with knowledge to give, but your students will teach you more than you teach them. If you want to truly master your art, teach it. Not when you're perfect. Not when you've figured everything out. Now. While you're still learning. Because teaching is how you learn what you actually know versus what you only think you know.

Teaching Formula

Knowledge is deep understanding. Not just the technique, but the why behind it. Why this stance and not that one? Why does the hip rotate before the hand extends? You need to know the technique, the principles that govern it, the common mistakes students make, the progressions to teach it effectively, and the applications where it's useful. Knowledge comes from curiosity and humility, from admitting what you don't know and going to find the answer.

Demonstration is where knowledge becomes visible. You must show it from multiple angles. Slow, then fast. With power, then with precision. The right way and the wrong way. But demonstration also means demonstrating the attitude you want your students to develop. If you show up late, they'll show up late. If you make excuses, they'll make excuses. Your discipline, your focus, your respect—all of it is on display every moment you're in front of students.

Repetition is the engine that turns knowledge and demonstration into skill. Start with the basic movement in isolation. Then add complexity—speed, power, combinations. Then add resistance—pads, sparring, competition. Each layer requires its own repetition. And here's the critical part: repetition must be monitored and corrected. *Bad repetition ingrains bad habits.*

Mastery is inevitable if you apply the formula correctly. Mastery means the student can execute the technique without thinking about it, can teach it to someone else, can apply it under pressure, and can recognize when not to use it.

Here's the gift that keeps on giving: every time you apply this formula to teaching, you're reinforcing it in yourself. You're deepening your knowledge by explaining it. You're sharpening your demonstration by performing it repeatedly. One organized ring fight is worth one hundred classes. One hour teaching a white belt is worth ten hours training alone. Why? Because teaching forces you through every level of mastery. You can't fake it. You get more out of doing less.

A great fighter picks apart their opponent, tests them, and finds the areas to attack where the opponent is weakest. These same skills in understanding people—reading capability, identifying vulnerability, exploiting weakness—are elements of what make a great teacher.

A student needs to know where they should apply their efforts. I start with working on and shoring up the weak points. If you cannot fix them completely, mask them. Then hone the strengths. Add value by identifying the weaknesses and strengths in others. The teacher gains experience in reading others and that can help your students improve both personally and by example for their future teaching style.

Look for your personal style, find your gifts and showcase them. Others will have to follow the same path to their own gifts. First they can see your obvious prowess and try to model it. After enough practice they will inherently mold what they are learning from you to meet their own gifts—a type of personal interpretation of what they have been taught. Then the knowledge becomes theirs, once it has been personalized, run through their own understanding and fit to their capabilities and particular physicality.

The more students you teach, the more patterns you recognize. Flexible students struggle with power generation. Heavy students struggle with speed and cardio. Timid students struggle with aggression. Athletic students struggle with patience and technique. Each type of student personality needs different coaching, different drills, different encouragement. The wider your range in managing students needs successfully, the better and more refined understanding you have in your own development.

Great teachers help students see their own strengths and weaknesses. You don't just tell them "your kicks are weak"—you show them. Film them. Compare their kicks to an advanced student's kicks. Break down the differences. Then create a specific plan: "You need more hip flexibility. Here's a stretching routine. Do it daily for a month. Let's test your kicks again and measure improvement." Specific. Measurable. Time-bound. This is how you build progress, not just activity.

Reading Your Students

After class, a trained instructor can tell you: who improved, who regressed, who's about to quit, and what each student needs next week. No guesswork here, only facts and reality recalled with maximum accuracy. It's pattern recognition built through attention and experience. Read your students like you've learned to read an opponent.

Watch for the physical tells. The student whose shoulders are creeping up toward their ears? They're tense, probably frustrated or scared. The one who's suddenly moving slower despite being early in class? Either injured or mentally checked out. The student who used to make eye contact but now stares at the floor? Something shifted. Find the fix for them in particular and learn something new about people in general.

Watch for the mental patterns. Who asks questions? That's

engagement. Who stops asking questions after weeks of asking them? That's either mastery or surrender—you need to figure out which. Who practices the technique between rounds while everyone else is resting? That's hunger.

Here's a technique that separates good instructors from great ones. You walk over to one student making a mistake. Physically correct the person who needs adjustment while giving the group the instruction on what to watch for and fix. Example, "After you extend, your hands should return to guard immediately." Everyone in the room is now checking their own hands because they saw you correct someone. The student you touched learned kinesthetically. The students watching learned visually. The students listening learned auditorily. Three different learning styles, taught, simultaneously.

Know who to correct publicly and who to correct privately. Some students thrive on public attention. Others shut down when singled out. You learn the difference by paying attention.

After every class, do your own debrief. Who improved today? Who's plateauing? Who looked like they might not come back? Reach out to that last one. A text message: "Good work today. See you next class." Sometimes that's all it takes.

How We Learn

In 1956, a psychologist named Benjamin Bloom asked a deceptively simple question: What does it actually mean to learn something?

His answer changed the way we look at educating people.

Bloom identified three distinct domains — three dimensions of the human learner. The first is cognitive: the world of knowledge, understanding, and thought. The second is affective: the inner world of values, emotion, and motivation — the part of you that decides whether something matters. And the third is psychomotor: the body, the hands, the muscle memory that turns knowledge into action.

Lets examine the three closer.

Think about it this way. A person who only develops the mind can describe exactly how to throw a punch — the mechanics, the physics, the angles — but cannot land one. A person who only develops the body can fight with instinct and power, but when something stops working, they have no idea why. And a person who only develops the heart? They have passion. They have fire. But without knowledge or skill to channel it, that fire burns without direction.

Real learning lives at the intersection of all three.

Bloom stressed, you cannot skip levels. Growth is sequential. A beginner needs to be shown, told, and shown again. They need explanation. They need patience. The intermediate learner needs to be challenged — put in the fire, then asked, what did you notice? The advanced learner needs something rarer still: the freedom to create, to question, to teach.

Which brings us to perhaps the most powerful idea in all of learning theory.

When you teach someone, you are forced to climb higher than them. You cannot guide a student through understanding unless you are already operating at analysis. You cannot lead someone through creation unless you are living at the level of evaluation. Teaching doesn't just transfer knowledge — it demands it. It pulls you upward.

The best learners, almost without exception, are also teachers.

Not because teaching is a gift they give to others — but because it's the fastest path to their own mastery.

Value of Tournaments

"The master has failed more times than the beginner has even tried." Steven McCranie. 2009

You want to know what kind of teacher you really are? Take your students to compete. Not to win. To fail in front of each other and learn that failure isn't death.

When you travel to a tournament with students, the dynamic changes. The familiar dojo is gone. The controlled environment vanishes. Now you're in a high school gym with bad lighting, other schools warming up with techniques you've never seen, and your students looking at you like you're supposed to have all the answers. This is where you learn to teach.

The techniques you drilled for months suddenly don't work because the referee is calling the match differently. The strategy you planned falls apart because your student drew the defending champion in the first round. The confidence you built evaporates when your student loses badly and comes off the mat crying.

The enlightenment comes in real time as you learn which techniques actually work under pressure. You learn which parts of your teaching stuck and which parts crumbled when tested. You learn that the student you thought was ready wasn't, and the student you underestimated just took third place against competitors twice their size.

Tournament travel also creates a bond that classroom training never will. You've spent twelve hours in a van together. You've watched each other lose, win, panic, recover. When you get home, training is different. The students who competed together have a shared reference point.

Tournament travel teaches you your program's weaknesses. If all your students struggle with the same thing under competition pressure, that's not their failure—it's yours. Maybe you're not drilling enough live scenarios. Maybe you're not teaching them how to manage adrenaline. You can ignore these lessons in the safety of your dojo. You can't ignore them when your student loses and asks you why the technique didn't work.

One organized tournament is worth a hundred classes of theoretical training. For your students, yes. But more importantly, for you.

To be successful in raising children or raising students, there is a similar process and system that can be utilized. S.M.A.R.T. goals are Specific, Measurable, Achievable, Relevant, and Time-bound.

Help your students distinguish between process goals and result goals:

Process Goals:

– Daily: I will train every day for one hour

– Weekly: I will spar twice a week with different part ers

– Monthly: I will learn a new form and perform it from memory

Result Goals:

– I want a black belt in four years

– I want to compete and place in the top three

– I want to master the spinning hook kick

The key is teaching students to picture "I want to" and "I get to" rather than "I have to." The language matters. "I have to train today" is obligation. "I get to train today" is privilege. Process goals are what you control. Results follow process. The student who trains consistently, who shows up four times a week, who drills techniques between classes—that student will achieve results.

When to Accept, When to Question

When you're a white belt, your job is simple: shut up and learn. You don't know enough to know what you don't know. You can't evaluate whether a technique is effective because you have zero reference point. So when your instructor tells you to do something that seems strange, do it anyway. Not because they're infallible, but because you're not qualified to judge yet.

Seek not to argue with your instructors. Your job at this

stage is absorption, not analysis. But pay attention internally. Watch what works for advanced students. Notice which techniques your instructor uses when they spar versus which ones they only utilize in drills. Don't argue about these observations—just collect them.

As you progress to intermediate levels, your questioning should shift. You're still executing what you're taught, but now you test variations privately. You try the technique in sparring to see if it holds up. If something consistently fails, now you can ask about it respectfully. Not "this technique doesn't work"—that's ego. But "I'm having trouble making this work against taller opponents. Can you show me what I'm missing?"

By the time you're advanced, you're operating at a level where you can have actual technical discussions with your instructor. You're developing your personal interpretation of the art. And sometimes, that means respectfully disagreeing with aspects of your instructor's approach. You can disagree with a technique while still practicing it out of respect for your instructor and the tradition.

When you become an instructor yourself, your job is to question everything internally—but not out loud to your students. Why am I teaching this? Is this the most effective method? You should be researching, experimenting, evolving. But you don't burden your white belts with your doubts.

The wisdom hierarchy:

– White Belt: Accept and execute. Questions for clarification only.

– Intermediate: Execute and observe. Questions about application.

– Advanced: Evaluate and discuss. Questions that advance understanding.

– Instructor: Examine and evolve. Questions for yourself.

Think of the current state of the students you are instructing. Imagine where you were when you were at their point in training. Think of all the questions you would have liked answered and then expect there will be surprise ones. You will need multiple ways of describing your answer to fully satisfy different student capabilities.

If you find yourself frustrated with the lack of progress of a student, take a breath and make a plan to address it. The frustration is often because your current plan is failing. The student isn't the problem—your approach to that student is the problem. Adjust. Try a different explanation. Give them a modified drill. Change something, because what you're doing isn't working.

Learning to teach means learning to see. You will encounter students spanning the entire spectrum of human capability—from natural athletes who could kill with their bare hands to gentle souls who must overcome deep psychological barriers just to imagine striking another person with force.

The revelation comes when you watch your least physically capable student—struggling with coordination, flexibility, or strength—pour maximum effort into every session while your most naturally gifted student coasts at seventy percent. Over time, you witness the struggling student transform through sheer determination while the gifted one stagnates through complacency.

Understanding arrives when you see why two students with vastly different capabilities can both earn a black belt. The belt doesn't measure absolute ability—it measures growth, commitment, and mastery relative to potential. One student may execute techniques with devastating power and flawless mechanics. Another may never achieve that level of physical prowess but has conquered fear, built discipline, and maximized every ounce of their capability.

Both deserve the belt. Both have achieved mastery. They simply started from different places on the mountain.

The question isn't "How capable are you now?" It's "How far have you traveled from where you began?" A student who started timid, uncoordinated, and weak but became confident, capable, and strong has completed an epic journey—even if their "strong" would be average for someone else.

This is why we evaluate effort, progress, and transformation, not just the final product in isolation. The black belt recognizes the journey as much as the destination.

Being a Mentor

As an instructor, you stand in an elevated role. The pedestal that lifts you to admiration also exposes you to judgment. You cannot press delete on what you teach—it becomes permanent in the lives you touch. This is both the weight and the privilege of the position. Teachers are remembered forever, so ask yourself: How do you want to be remembered?

Strive to embody the ideals you held for your own instructors, then surpass them. Live up to the best version of what a teacher should be, knowing that even touching one life creates a lasting legacy.

Beyond Technique

Mentorship extends far beyond teaching kicks and submissions. Your role is to guide students through the entire journey—the training, yes, but also the mental struggles that define growth. The doubt that whispers "quit." The plateau that tests persistence. The injury that demands patience. The loss that exposes weakness. The competition anxiety that reveals the gap between preparation and readiness.

Your job isn't to remove these obstacles. It's to reframe them as essential parts of the path. The injury teaches body awareness. The loss teaches humility. The plateau reveals that growth isn't linear. The doubt forces deliberate recommitment. These aren't problems to solve—they're lessons to absorb.

Students need to know they're not alone in these moments. Every black belt felt the same way. The instructor they admire wanted to quit multiple times but didn't. The struggle they're experiencing is normal, expected, and survivable. Your honesty about your own journey gives them permission to struggle and keep going.

Translating Experience Into Wisdom

A great mentor shows students where to look, but not what to see. You've amassed years of experience—training, competing, failing, succeeding, getting hurt, overcoming. Your intelligence deciphers that experience into wisdom. You compress years of trial and error into lessons absorbed in minutes, saving your students from mistakes you made by teaching them what those mistakes revealed.

But remember: the strongest people are often the most sensitive. Those who show the most kindness are frequently the first to be mistreated. Those who care for everyone else usually need care the most. As you pour yourself into your students, recognize their struggles—family problems, health issues, job stress, the weight of existence that no one escapes. Your awareness and compassion during their hard times may matter more than any technique you teach.

Building Community

Remind your students constantly that their mission is to help each other to learn, and grow together. Respect for training partners builds a team atmosphere where everyone elevates everyone else. A rising tide lifts all boats. When students improve through their own effort, that improvement magnifies tenfold when united with their teacher's effort and the support within their training community.

Teaching is Training

"When it comes to training, I do that through teaching."—

MATTHEW BLACK

Ryron Gracie, 2004

I have always seen myself as the perpetual student. Seeking out experts and looking to far off schools for the ultimate techniques and sage masters for secret wisdoms. Oddly, it seems I learn as much or more when I give my time to advance others. I have found that when I teach basics I find new ways of incorporating the movements into more applications. By examining the fundamentals with students, I perfect the skill in my own repertoire. Training those seeking to learn is among the most rewarding functions in this lifetime. Teaching requires balance: deep understanding of your craft and how you execute it forms one half; how you transmit that knowledge forms the other. Only when you've achieved authority over your own actuality—when you've become a master of yourself—can you truly grow by reaching out to help others achieve the same capability.

Your teaching becomes immortal when it lives in your students. They carry it forward, adapt it, improve upon it, and pass it on. A diamond forever cherished, polished and heirloomed. Your contributions become part of a lineage stretching back centuries that will continue long after you're gone. This is the true legacy: not the techniques you taught, but the lives you shaped and the chain of knowledge you strengthened.

A teacher's job is to lead by example. Your students don't need perfection from you. They need authenticity. They need to see someone who has walked the path, who continues to train diligently, who embodies the principles they're trying to teach. To your students, you are the living manifestation of the Martial Arts.

Teaching is the final polish. It's where you discover what you truly know and what you only thought you knew. It's where your understanding becomes wisdom. It's where your journey becomes a map for others. And in showing them the way, you see the path more clearly yourself.

Your Next Step

If you're already teaching: Recommit. Look at your students with fresh eyes. Ask yourself if you're giving them your best —not your perfect, but your authentic best. Train with them, struggle alongside them, and let them see that the journey never ends, even for the instructor.

If you're not yet teaching: Consider it. You don't need to be a master to share what you know. You simply need to be a few steps ahead on the path and willing to reach back for those behind you. Start small—help a junior student with a technique, offer encouragement to someone struggling, share one lesson you've learned. Teaching begins the moment you decide someone else's progress matters as much as your own.

The martial arts survive because knowledge flows forward. You received instruction from someone who received it from someone before them, stretching back through generations. Now the chain reaches you. Will you pass it on? Will you become the teacher someone remembers forever?

The dojo is waiting. Your students—current or future—are waiting. The only question left is: What kind of teacher will you choose to be?

CHAPTER 15 – PURIFY THE WARRIOR

"The only reason a warrior is alive is to fight, and the only reason a warrior fights is to win."— Miyamoto Musashi, A Book of Five Rings. 1645

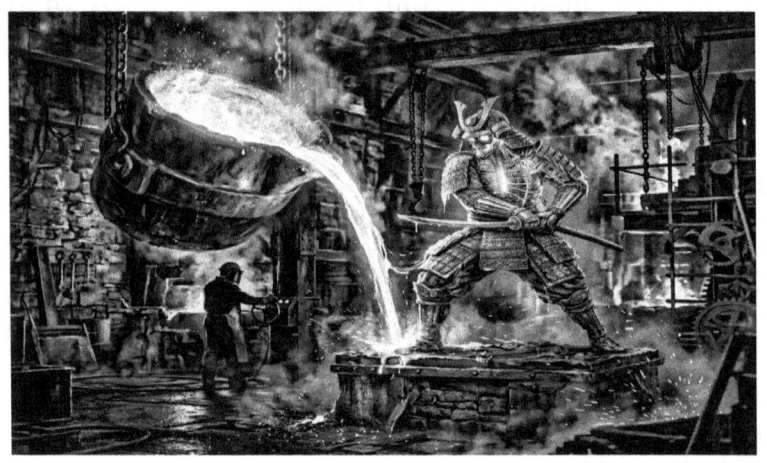

Fighting does not make one a warrior. It is not about the fight, it is about what you fight for. A warrior fights for what is right. A warrior harmonizes and marinates inside this state of mind and attitude, always preparing and expecting the fight, a practical person who realizes having his shoes tied and double knotted may save his life.

Once you have trained and can be considered a martial artist by your peers, 80% of the work is done. This chapter is to advise you about your continuing journey on the path. Now it is time to polish and refine yourself. First and foremost, your challenge is to be ready for the fight, anytime and anywhere. Secondly, to be mindful on your role as an example to others and to properly fulfill the function of the warrior class in society. This is a heavy burden and many around you will come to rely on you to be the bedrock of their defense. Feeling, unmotivated? Tired? Sick? Drinking? Injured? Too bad. Anytime for any reason, because often by surprise, the fight picks you.

Find a Warrior's Balance

"Wen Wu Shuang Quan" (文武双全) This concept means "accomplished in both the pen and the sword." Chinese warrior-scholars were expected to master both martial arts and the "Four Arts" (琴棋書畫): music (particularly the guqin), strategy games (like Go), calligraphy, and painting. Confucian philosophy held that true excellence required both civil and military accomplishment. Many famous generals were also renowned poets and calligraphers.

You need this too. Train hard. Fight hard. But also cultivate something beautiful, something peaceful, something that reminds you why you're training in the first place. Expand your mind otherwise the parts not exercised atrophy.

I've seen fighters who only train aggression become brittle—unable to relax, unable to recover, burning out from constant intensity. The ones who last, the ones who grow old in the art without breaking, understand balance.

All Warrior Codes Agree

Similarly to Chinese generals and the Japanese samurai, medieval knights under the code of chivalry were expected to be educated in music, poetry, dance, and courtly manners. The ideal knight wasn't just a brutal warrior but a **refined gentleman**—skilled in falconry, chess, and composing romantic poetry. The concept of the "Renaissance man" later evolved from this, exemplified by figures like Leonardo da Vinci who was both engineer and artist.

Find your art. Find what centers you when the darkness gets too close. Because it will. The things you'll see, the things you'll do, the things done to you—these leave marks. Art doesn't erase them, but it reminds you that beauty exists alongside brutality. That you contain multitudes. That you are more than your capacity for violence. The goal is not just to be dangerous. It is to be complete.

Black Belt Is Just the Beginning

You've seen it happen. A student trains for years—blood, sweat, frustration, breakthroughs, setbacks—and finally earns their black belt. Everyone celebrates. Photos are taken. Congratulations pour in.

Then what?

Some students think they've arrived. They treat the black belt like a finish line. They coast. They stop growing. They stop trying and eventually stop training.

They've completely misunderstood what the black belt means.

The black belt actually represents the phase of training where you may officially take on the responsibility of adapting the art to you. It is the recognized standard that you understand the fundamentals and have proven proficiency in them. You now may take them and make them your own. Use the basic methods and the core structure as taught, but now the artist in you can shine through.

The black belt isn't the end—**it's permission to begin.** Being a martial artist is meant to be permanent, to continue for your lifetime.

Everything before black belt is learning the alphabet. Now you can string the letters together and create prose and poetry.

You've mastered the building blocks and functional basics

well enough to begin expressing them in ways unique to your body, your style, your understanding. This is where you stop being a student mimicking techniques and start becoming an artist creating your own expression of the art.

Danger of Success

Once you've become a true warrior, never lose your drive for cultivation. Many have fallen to their own success—content and complacent with levels achieved, with no external threats to sharpen them, they got caught up in drugs, pride, or the assertion of power over others.

Nietzsche warned us: *In times of peace, a warlike man attacks himself.* Without something to struggle against, a warrior turns inward and wages war on himself or those in their intimate circle. He also cautioned: *"Whoever fights monsters should see to it that in the process he does not become a monster himself."* The restless energy of someone who spent years building the ability to defend against all comers will be tempted to use that power—becoming jaded or prideful and no longer seeking the monster but attacking friends and allies; transforming into the monster he had originally trained to defeat.

Here is the trap. Success breeds comfort. Comfort breeds complacency. Complacency breeds death. The warrior must resist the siren call of "enough." There is no enough. There is only the next challenge, the next refinement, the next purification.

Mind Altering Substances

Psychological operations are the most expensive line item in global military budgets. Spanning peace and wartime, psyops and drug wars are waged nonstop by national intelligence agencies—internally and externally. **This is a grave threat to the warrior class.** If it wasn't, these wouldn't still be the number one fracturing tool in conquests from time immemorial. It is a strategy of turning the *warlike man against himself* through addiction, and the wider spin off effects of inebriation. Society loses cohesiveness when its protectors are drunks.

My advice? **Do not drink or do drugs.** Altering your state—even slightly—softens even the toughest person. Step into the ring knowing your opponent defiles his integrated being with unclean habits and drinking, and you instantly have the upper hand. No matter how hard he trains, these habits erase some of that effort and results.

Why? Because alcohol and drugs have always been weapons of war. Alcohol was prohibited and still is in many countries because, like any addiction, it can be weaponized. War is waged first on the mind long before the physical battle begins. History proves this: the Opium Wars, firewater distributed to North American natives, and countless other conquests. Taking drugs creates distraction, and it's dangerously easy to need distractions at an accelerating rate until you are permanently distracted. That is not the path of the warrior. That is not a condition in which a warrior can thrive. Do not fall victim to unconventional, asymmetric, non kinetic weapons of war.

The same principle applies to unnecessary pharmaceuticals. Do not take painkillers like Tylenol or aspirin unless absolutely necessary. There are fewer safety controls on "over-the-counter" drugs than prescription drugs, and evidence shows they wreak havoc on your kidneys and liver—even worse than alcohol. Suffering through pain builds your natural tolerance. One day you may really need the full benefit of these drugs, and it's better if you're a lightweight requiring very little to be effective.

And pornography? Absolute poison for the mind—the same as any powerful drug. The CIA distributed free pornography before and throughout the war in Iraq in what was considered a successful operation. This is another commonly used military psyop tool, designed to fracture focus, hijack reward systems, and corrupt intimate bonds. Stay away from it altogether and preserve your mental health and your intimate relations.

The warrior's mind is the ultimate weapon. Protect it.

Face Reality

The fight still lies ahead. The challenges come in all forms: bullies and dictators, illness and accidents. The world is unfair, with everyone competing for resources and trying to get ahead. Those in charge are often dangerous. There's no guarantee of justice, and luck plays a big role—so create your own luck.

Living with honor, disciplined work ethic, self-respect, and healthy habits—applying all the principles in this book—will tilt favor to your benefit. Take an active hand in directing your future. Try, then try harder, then do it again with more vigor. Push until you bleed. And if you die, die doing what was worthwhile.

No one is coming to save you. **Take personal responsibility**. It is your fight, your cross to bear. Every day, with intention, engage life head-on. Shirk this duty at your peril.

It is not pessimism—it's realism. The world doesn't care about your feelings, your excuses, your reasons. It only responds to action, strength, and will. So become strong. Become willful. Take action. Every single day.

Know Your Why

Life delivers experiences that through contemplation form your personal philosophy. Your basic beliefs, values, concepts, and attitudes are brought to light by evaluating and answering your "why." To check what's foundational to you, explain confidently why you're doing what you're doing with your life.

For deeper insight, **expand the "why" line of questioning**. Many don't take time to search themselves for these reasons—

some haven't even considered them. Many cannot explain why they do what they do each day. Understanding your "why" and firmly owning what guides your decisions is essential for confident life choices and provides conscious control over your life's direction.

You'll be most satisfied when you have a thinking hand in directing your life rather than taking a back seat and being swayed in random directions without your input at the wheel.

Build on Truth

To be considered peaceful, you must be capable of extreme violence. If you're not capable of violence, you're not peaceful—you're harmless. There's a difference. Make yourself fully capable, then seek total peace. Dangerously peaceful, not harmlessly peaceful.

Honesty and discipline are fundamental to a warrior. Without honesty, you build on sand. Without discipline, you cannot maintain what you've built. These two pillars hold up everything else. Compromise them and the entire structure collapses. A warrior who lies to himself is already defeated before the first blow is thrown.

Once you commit to building your life on truth, the next step is learning to work with reality as it actually is—not as you wish it were.

Accept Reality

Find the challenge in everything and accept it with a smile and a spring in your step. The saying "Life sucks, get a helmet" captures an important truth: the norm of human existence is chaos and things going wrong.

Picture this: Your sparring partner catches you with a clean shot to the ribs—hard enough that you'll feel it tomorrow. Most people would back off, make excuses, or let frustration take over. But you've trained for this moment. You smile, touch gloves, and reset your mind. That sharp pain isn't a setback; it's data. Your guard dropped when you committed to that hook. Now you know.

This is the difference: the untrained mind sees the hit as punishment and wants to quit. The martial artist sees it as tuition—you just paid for a lesson you'll never forget. While your opponent hopes to discourage you, you're already adjusting, already improving. They gave you exactly what you needed: a challenge to accept, a weakness to fix, and proof that you can take a hit and keep moving forward.

That's not just about fighting. That's about life. The job rejection, the failed business, the relationship that didn't work—those are all clean shots to the ribs. You can either protect yourself from ever trying again, or you can smile, touch gloves with reality, and get back in the ring with better defense.

Expect the worst, hope for the best, and you'll be well-adjusted and positive—because you understand the norm is for things not to work out, that you don't have total control, and it's pretty darn nice when things work in your favor. When things go right, celebrate it.

Life doesn't get easier as a martial artist—but you forge the tools to face the toughest challenges. This separates warriors from everyone else. While others complain about difficulty, you greet it head-on. While others seek comfort, you seek the hard road.

And that brings us to perhaps the most counter-intuitive principle of warrior philosophy: the shortcut is always the longest path.

Less is More; Take the Hard Road

Shortcuts end up being the longest road. Do not cut corners. If you want something badly, work hard for it, and no one will be able to take it away from you. Always take the hard narrow road—the flat wide avenue leads to ruin.

Here's the formula for true success: Work hard. Do what is

right. Don't shortcut or cheat. Your time will come.

When faced with a challenge or decision, identify which choice is the easy way out—then do the opposite. Whether it involves money, training, a loved one, or a friend, if you do the hardest thing, you'll always be more satisfied with the result. Sacrifice has its own reward. There is wisdom in the austere. Those who do more with less present themselves without worry about material things. The less you have, the more you can focus on what really matters. Meditate on this.

Let me give you a concrete example of this principle in action.

Consider the white belt who shows up at 5 AM for open mat while his training partners sleep in. He's exhausted. His body aches from yesterday's session. The easy choice is obvious: hit snooze, skip one day, no one will notice. But he doesn't take it. He drives through the dark, steps onto the mat before sunrise, and drills his fundamentals—alone—while the rest of the world chooses comfort.

Six months later, that same white belt earns his blue belt ahead of students who started before him. A year later, he's the one newer students watch and want to emulate. But here's what matters more than the belt: he knows what he's made of. When life demands he show up exhausted—for a sick parent, a struggling business, a relationship worth fighting for—he already knows he can do it. He's already proven it to himself a hundred times on the mat at 5 AM.

The students who slept in? They're still white belts, wondering why progress feels so slow. They took the flat, wide, lackadaisical avenue and found it led nowhere. He took the hard, narrow road—and it forged him into someone who can't be broken by inconvenience.

Now, having built yourself through truth, reality, and hard work, **you're ready to tackle the most sophisticated challenge: solving problems in a way that elevates everyone in-**

volved.

Seek Win-Win-Win Solutions

Most people struggle to find even a simple compromise. A true win-win—where both parties genuinely benefit—is already considered masterful negotiation. Now consider the warrior's approach: the win-win-win. The best result possible.

This is the realm of exceptional problem-solving. Where two wins would already demonstrate skill, you're searching for three. Where most would celebrate finding common ground between two parties, you're engineering a solution that also serves the broader good, the long-term outcome, or a third party affected by the decision.

Start each day with the mantra of doing your best in all things. In situations where you have decisive power, train yourself to see beyond the obvious bilateral solution. Ask: "Who else is affected? What's the long-term impact? Is there a way everyone walks away better than they came?"

This requires deep meditation on problems. The lazy mind stops at the first acceptable answer. The disciplined mind keeps searching: Can you satisfy both immediate parties AND create a positive ripple effect? Can you meet today's needs AND improve tomorrow's conditions? Can you serve individual interests AND strengthen the collective?

Let me be clear—not everyone will be completely happy. Perfect satisfaction for all is often impossible. But in balance, no one should feel victimized by your actions. More importantly, when you achieve a genuine win-win-win, you've done something rare. You've found the elegant solution that most people never see because they stopped looking after "good enough." This is a case where a warrior can become a peace maker and avoid a war for the benefit of all involved. What is the saying? Peacemakers will inherit the earth? Perhaps because the war-makers disappear through mutual destruction.

A warrior always seeks to excel. If you put in the effort and actually find a win for everyone involved—the immediate parties, the organization, the long-term outcome—that's a great accomplishment. This is leadership thinking. This is strategic mastery. The world would be a much better place if everyone operated at this level, but few will. The fact that it's difficult is precisely why it's worth pursuing.

Self-Discipline Builds Warriors

The best warriors are built through self-discipline. Once you've mastered a martial art, you'll have a guide and mental edge on others around you. You'll understand the gravity of setting a goal and know how to stick with it. Anything can be achieved once your mind is made up and your will is strong. You'll have learned to overcome struggles and obstacles, to face your fears.

The deeper truth? **The real opponent was always you.** The version of you that wanted to quit, that made excuses, that chose comfort over growth. Martial arts doesn't just teach you to fight—it teaches you that you're capable of defeating the weakest parts of yourself. And once you've done that in training, you can do it anywhere: at 11 PM when you need to finish the project, at 5 AM when the run feels impossible, in the conversation where apologizing feels like losing.

The techniques will fade if you don't practice them. The muscle will atrophy if you don't use it. But the person you became in the process of mastering them—disciplined, resilient, honest about your limitations—that stays with you. That's the real weapon you've forged. Not a punch or a kick, but a mind that doesn't flinch when difficulty arrives. A character that treats "I can't" as a question, not an answer.

Most people go through life hoping they have what it takes. You'll know you do—because you've already tested yourself in the crucible and refused to break.

Multiple Attackers

Don't train to match others—train to exceed yourself, like the **Ninja on the Mountain.** A mob is always weaker than its numbers suggest. Ten men charging together aren't ten independent warriors—they're a hive mind, attacking on command, retreating on instinct, moving without conviction. They have no individual center. *Ōsensei* (the great teacher) Ueshiba, the founder of Aikido, saw this:

> *"Even though surrounded by several enemies, fight with the thought that they are but one." — Morihei Ueshiba, 1968*

Because they are one—one collective cowardice pretending to be strength. They attack together because none of them would attack alone. They follow orders, not truth. But you? You've trained to impress yourself, not to match the group. You operate from your own center, your own standard, your own will. That makes you whole. That makes them fragmented.

The warrior who answers only to himself will always defeat the crowd that answers to each other.

This same illusion plays out in boardrooms and office politics.

You present an idea that challenges the status quo. Suddenly, five colleagues who never agreed on anything are united against you. The VP piles on. HR sends a "concerned" email. Someone whispers that you're "not a team player." It feels like you're surrounded.

But look closer. They're not five independent thinkers who each evaluated your proposal and found it lacking. They're one scared organism protecting itself from change. They attack together because the group gives them permission to do what none of them would risk alone. They're following the unspoken command: *preserve comfort, eliminate threat.*

This is spiritual combat, and the same principle applies. The mob has no center. They derive their confidence from each other, which means they have no confidence at all. The moment you refuse to flinch, the moment you stand on your own truth without needing their validation, the illusion shatters. They'll sense it. One will waver. Then another. The hive mind can't sustain itself against someone who isn't afraid of being alone.

You've trained for this. Every time you showed up when it was easier to quit, every time you held your standard when others lowered theirs, you were preparing for exactly this moment. You don't need the group's approval because you've already earned your own.

The warrior who knows his own center cannot be moved by a crowd that has none.

Continue to Train Like It's Real

Always train to the level you know you can perform in your heart, mind, and soul. Do it because you're sure you could do it if REALLY pushed. Train to impress yourself. Your self respect will grow. Even if your days of being deployed are over and you are settled in a retired or teaching role, train with the intensity like you might be outside the wire tomorrow. You may have trained for years to be in this position, but this is no time to slack off. Stay chiseled, stay focused and live up to your legacy. Leadership should shine brightly to be the light for all who would follow.

Being well-trained carries a dangerous side effect: overconfidence. Never boast or grow too proud—it's guaranteed to make you look a fool. Many fighters reach a point where they overestimate themselves and underestimate others. This is a sure path to losing fights. A well-rounded warrior has perhaps a 30% advantage over the untrained, and only 5% over those wise in the martial ways. The margins are thinner than ego wants to believe.

The Rabbit and the Fox

I have always assumed my opponent is a better all-around combatant than myself, then set out to prove him wrong. By assuming they're better, I weaken their position—I'm already the underdog, fighting for my life rather than my pride. I know I am not the only one to approach fighting this way.

Consider the parable of the rabbit and the fox: The fox rarely beats the rabbit in a race because the rabbit runs for its very life, while the fox is only running for its lunch. This describes the level of commitment required in every encounter. Practice this method of feverous defense and offense, and you will win with the rabbit's odds.

Grandmaster Lee Said

When I received my green belt, I started working as a nightclub bouncer to test my skills in real situations. My Grandmaster asked if I wanted to know the secret to being the best fighter in the world. I said yes. He told me: ***Don't fight.*** In this way, you cannot be beaten and will have an unblemished record.

The answer seemed like a letdown at the time, but it served me well. From then on, I stopped taking every inferred challenge and every fight opportunity that presented itself. Strategic avoidance is not cowardice—it's wisdom.

Build Your Army

Do your part to build your community. Be a contributor and a person of value to all those around you. The saying goes: be kind to strangers, you never know when you are in the company of angels. I've met complete strangers who helped me through tough situations with genuine kindness and wholehearted giving. The most admired martial artists in history were champions of their neighborhoods, with loyal fans following them for entire careers.

Pay it forward before you ever need to ask a favor. **Humility is the hallmark of the true warrior**, and service is the ultimate understanding of his role in this existence. Volunteer. Give warmly to charities with both time and money. Giving money is easy—giving time is more valuable and meaningful, both for others and yourself. True character develops in the lowliest of tasks.

You may one day face a threat requiring many allies to defeat—an unscrupulous boss, a corrupt official, an overwhelming adversary. With your history of selfless investment in others, you will find many who rally to your cause. This is combat at the highest level: recruiting others to fight alongside you for friendship, love, honor, respect, and loyalty. You are building your own loyal army.

Think for Yourself

Come to all your own conclusions. Make all your biases your own. Unlearn anything you've been told and find the truth as best you can understand it. Take ownership of all your thoughts, opinions, and actions. When you apply critical thought with an open mind, you act according to your highest level of effort to be correct.

You will not rely on other people's opinions, research, or manipulation. You will decide based on your highest level of thinking with as much information as can be gathered. But don't become so attached to an idea that you cannot separate yourself from it. **You are not your ideas**—don't hang your ego on them.

A true warrior questions everything, including himself. *Especially* himself.

Eloquent Wish

Rudyard Kipling wrote a poem in 1910. It describes the character we're building through martial discipline. Read it. Memorize it. Live it.

If—Rudyard Kipling

If you can keep your head when all about you
Are losing theirs and blaming it on you,
If you can trust yourself when all men doubt you,
But make allowance for their doubting too;
If you can wait and not be tired by waiting,
Or being lied about, don't deal in lies,
Or being hated, don't give way to hating,
And yet don't look too good, nor talk too wise:
If you can dream—and not make dreams your master;
If you can think—and not make thoughts your aim;
If you can meet with Triumph and Disaster
And treat those two impostors just the same;
If you can bear to hear the truth you've spoken
Twisted by knaves to make a trap for fools,
Or watch the things you gave your life to, broken,
And stoop and build 'em up with worn-out tools:
If you can make one heap of all your winnings
And risk it on one turn of pitch-and-toss,
And lose, and start again at your beginnings
And never breathe a word about your loss;
If you can force your heart and nerve and sinew
To serve your turn long after they are gone,
And so hold on when there is nothing in you
Except the Will which says to them: 'Hold on!'
If you can talk with crowds and keep your virtue,
Or walk with Kings—nor lose the common touch,
If neither foes nor loving friends can hurt you,
If all men count with you, but none too much;
If you can fill the unforgiving minute
With sixty seconds' worth of distance run,
Yours is the Earth and everything that's in it,
  And—which is more—you'll be a Man, my son!

This poem captures the essence of this chapter. I want it

to describe you. Holding on to a youthful exuberance for life, and having the humility and inner peace that balance brings. Keeping your head under pressure. **Trusting yourself despite doubt.** Meeting triumph and disaster with the same steady temperament. Forcing yourself to continue when you have nothing left except will. The warrior's code distilled into verse, yet it wasn't written for warriors or to warriors, it is written as hope for the betterment of every person who has walked the earth.

The "unforgiving minute" Kipling speaks of is every minute of your life. Each one demands sixty seconds of maximum effort, of distance run, of progress made. The minutes don't care about your excuses. They don't wait for you to feel ready. They pass whether you fill them with purpose or waste them with comfort. The warrior fills every unforgiving minute with intentional action.

Final Polish

The warrior must continue to purify and distill, to temper and sanctify themselves. Always in pursuit of a better version. This relentless pursuit is a lonely road because it must be traveled despite the lure to rest, to relax and accept the current state. No human can give 100% in relative terms all the time, only 100% of what we have available, but we can always give more than we are currently.

Slow and steady wins the race. If you train every day, you will reach your goals sooner than you think. The hardest part to any journey is the first step. There is no magic pill to make us who we desire to be overnight. We must form the plan and then put in the hard work to achieve it and make it our own.

A great warrior spends his life working on his entire being. Finding any flaw and repairing it, polishing his character, prestige and respect. A true warrior seeks every opportunity to build his courage so that he may face his death with bravery and honor.

This is the path. Not comfortable, not easy, but yours. Walk it with purpose. Walk it alone if you must. Walk it until you can walk no more, and then crawl. The warrior's journey never ends because perfection is impossible, but the pursuit of it is what defines us.

You are being forged. Every day, every challenge, every moment you choose the hard road over the easy one. The fire never goes out. Stay in it. Let it burn away everything that is not essential. What remains is the warrior, purified.

"Out of every 100 men, 10 should not be here,
80 are nothing but targets, 9 are the real fighters,
and we are lucky to have them, for they the battle make."
"Ah, but the ONE, ONE of them is a WARRIOR,
and he will bring the others back."
— Heraclitus, 500 BC

Be the ONE. And bring the others with you.

CHAPTER 16 – SUCCESS BREEDS SUCCESS

"The medicine for my suffering I had within me from the very beginning, but I did not take it. My ailment came from within myself, but I did not observe it until this moment. Now I see that I will never find the light unless, like the candle, I am my own fuel."—Bruce Lee, 1969

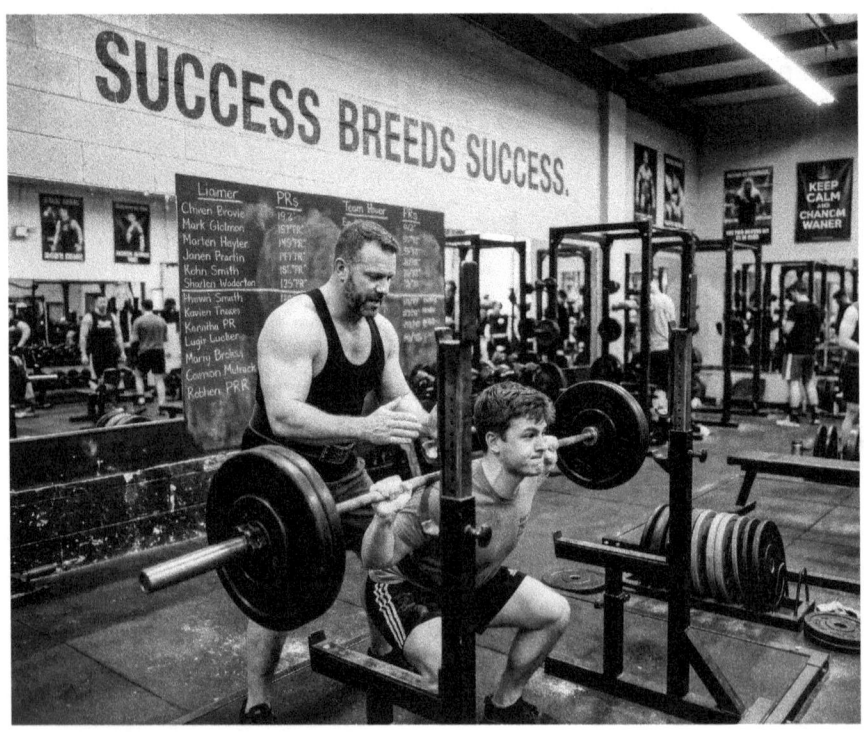

The Diamond You Have

Your keys to success are already inside of you. Following the martial path, you will learn how to wield them. At times you already are the scholar, the lover, and the warrior. The goal to consistently be these three people simultaneously is within your grasp. All you need is discipline and the willingness to never give up the fight to better yourself. Success in any arena is the result of predictable and consistent outcomes.

A diamond starts as a rough stone buried deep, holding extraordinary potential that no one can see. In its natural state, it's unremarkable—dull, unimpressive, easily overlooked. It takes a master craftsman to recognize what lies beneath the surface and the skill to reveal it. The jeweller doesn't create the diamond's value; it was always there. But without cutting, grinding, and polishing, that value remains hidden and worthless.

Each facet must be cut at precise angles, requiring patience, expertise, and countless hours of focused work. One facet alone does little. But as each new surface is carefully shaped and polished, the stone begins to catch light differently. The more facets added, the more brilliantly it sparkles, transforming from rough potential into something that captures attention and commands respect.

Each edge represents a difficult task accomplished—honed through hard work, careful planning, and precise execution. You are both the raw diamond and the master craftsman. The potential is already within you, but the refinement is your responsibility.

Success begins as an idea that is conceptualized, an attractive ambition. Your mind is an unparalleled machine—it just needs you to program it for the output you want. Discipline and clear intention to reach your objective are the foundational principles of all martial arts. They contain a whole of life strategy for achieving any goal you desire. You are a diamond in the rough, full of potential. Find your art and get the best of you to shine through.

And just as a diamond has many facets, so too does the complete human being.

Three Facets

Within each of us live three undeveloped archetypes: the scholar, the lover, and the warrior. These aren't just abstract concepts—they're real capacities that shape how effectively we move through life. Let me explain what each one represents and why you need all three.

The scholar seeks knowledge, understanding, and wisdom. This is the part of you that pursues truth through study and contemplation. Think of the researcher who stays up late reading, the professional who constantly upgrades their skills, the person who asks "why?" and "how?" until they truly understand. The scholar in you craves learning, values accuracy, and builds expertise through careful observation and analysis. Without the scholar, you operate on assumptions and instinct alone, never developing the depth of understanding that separates the novice from the master.

The lover embodies passion, connection, and creativity. This archetype represents your capacity for deep relationships, appreciation of beauty, and emotional depth. Picture the parent who connects with their children on a soul level, the artist who creates something that moves people to tears, the friend who truly sees and understands you. The lover in you feels deeply, creates bonds, and experiences the richness of human connection. Without the lover, life becomes mechanical and hollow—all achievement with no meaning, all progress with no joy.

The warrior represents discipline, courage, and action. This is the will to face challenges, protect what matters, and persist against resistance. Imagine the entrepreneur who launches their business despite fear, the athlete who trains when motivation is gone, the person who stands up for what's right even when it costs them something. The warrior in you takes what the scholar has learned and what the lover values, and fights to make it real in the world. Without the warrior, you're all knowledge and feeling with no ability to execute, to defend, to persevere when things get hard.

Now here's the problem many people face: They favor one or two of these aspects while neglecting the others, creating an imbalanced personality that struggles in certain domains of life.

Consider the brilliant intellectual who can explain complex theories but cannot connect emotionally with their own spouse or children. They have the scholar fully developed but the lover remains dormant. They achieve professional success but come home to empty relationships, wondering why their knowledge doesn't translate to happiness. Their family doesn't need another lecture—they need presence, warmth, emotional availability. But the scholar without the lover cannot provide this.

Or think about the passionate artist who pours their heart into creative work but lacks the discipline to finish projects, market their art, or build a sustainable career. They have the lover awakened but the warrior sleeps. They feel everything intensely, create beautiful moments, but cannot translate that passion into consistent action. Their work remains scattered in notebooks and unfinished canvases because they never developed the warrior's capacity to show up daily, to push through resistance, to do the unglamorous work that turns potential into reality.

Then there's the driven competitor who sacrifices relationships and learning in the pursuit of achievement. They have the warrior dominant but have neglected both scholar and lover. They're relentless in pursuit of goals, but those goals lack depth because they never took time to truly understand what they're building or why it matters. They win competitions but lose marriages. They climb the corporate ladder but arrive at the top alone, hollow, wondering why success feels so empty. The warrior without the scholar and lover becomes a machine—effective but soulless.

But the most complete human personality emerges when all three operate simultaneously in harmony.

This is the person who learns deeply, loves fully, and acts decisively. They study their craft with scholarly dedication, approach their relationships with a lover's passion, and pursue their goals with a warrior's discipline. They don't toggle between these modes—they integrate them. When facing a challenge at work, they bring the scholar's analysis, the lover's care for people affected by their decisions, and the warrior's courage to act despite uncertainty. This is the leader people want to follow. This is the partner people want to build a life with. This is the competitor others respect even in defeat.

Martial arts training is uniquely designed to develop all three facets simultaneously. The scholar emerges as you study techniques, learn your body's mechanics, and understand the philosophy behind the movements. The lover awakens as you build bonds with training partners, appreciate the beauty of a perfectly executed form, and connect with the lineage of masters who came before you. The warrior is forged through daily discipline, facing your fears in sparring, and persisting when every muscle screams to quit.

The art polishes all three facets of your diamond until each one catches the light and illuminates the others.

Expect Success

The rough uncut diamond is within you, your intrinsic internal value— Finding external value means recognizing it around you and setting a goal to get it. There's a saying: "Dress for success." To me that means to be so certain of yourself, that you fully invest in your guaranteed future success. Committing to your goals without reservation. Prepare as if your aspirations are all but achieved. Go out and buy a safe for your future cash, gold and silver coins. Build a trophy case for upcoming medals, ribbons, and accolades. Expect it, plan it, and commit to filling them both. Pretty embarrassing to have an empty trophy case? You know what to do. Know the destination, know the journey.

The Winner's Mindset

All of life is a struggle for resources and advancement. Some make winning look easy. Luck is always a factor, but consistent winners over the long term have systems and discipline that move the odds in their favor. Winners win because they employ time-tested systems with high probabilities for success. For many, that proven system is found in the martial arts. A vast majority of the worlds wealthy include martial training with the best coaches as part of their day. They don't advertise it, but then again, they don't explain how they got wealthy very specifically either. They have the formula and all you need to do is copy it for your own version of success.

IQ

Life is a psychology test that separates winners from the lazy and incompetent. The questions you face aren't the same as others, but they aren't that different either. You're handed a problem and asked to solve it. Over and over, you decide your own fate as you rise to the occasion, learn from mistakes, and see the patterns in your life and others' lives. Or you don't, and you're doomed to repeat the same failed tests. We can't beat what we don't understand. This is the scholar within you—the facet of your diamond that must be cut first because without it, you're swinging blind.

High IQ is described as quickly processing challenges and devising solutions. The quicker that process, the higher the score. But raw intelligence is like an uncut diamond—impressive potential that means nothing without refinement. You need more than the scholar's ability to analyze. You need the warrior's discipline to act decisively under pressure and the lover's intuition to read situations beyond pure logic. Intelligence alone isn't enough—we need battle-tested tools like the OODA loop as a guide. We need a firm emotional foundation from which to make critical decisions that tilt the scales between winning and losing, pleasure and pain, life and death. Each real-world problem you solve cuts another facet into your diamond. Each mistake you learn from polishes the surface. The martial artist understands that knowledge without application is worthless, and speed of thought without clarity of action gets you killed.

The Compound Effect

It is the combination of all of the teachings in martial arts that breed success. Success isn't a single achievement—it's a chain reaction. Like a stone dropped in still water, each new understanding of the underlying lesson creates ripples that generate the next wave of opportunities. The martial artist who trains with discipline doesn't just get stronger—they build confidence. That confidence doesn't just improve their fighting—it transforms how they carry themselves in the world. That presence they exude doesn't just command respect—it opens doors that were previously invisible. Each level unlocks the next.

This is the compound effect, and it's why martial arts training is one of the most valuable investments you can make in yourself. You're not just learning to fight. You're building a foundation that elevates every aspect of your existence. Success compounds on success.

A Cascade in Action

Here's where the compound effect becomes visible: The martial artist who has drilled techniques ten thousand times can observe an attack and act almost instantaneously—their orient and decide phases happen in milliseconds because they've compressed them through training. This faster OODA loop doesn't just make you a better fighter—it makes you better at everything.

In business, you read market shifts before competitors finish analyzing last quarter's data. In relationships, you sense tension and address it before it becomes conflict. In crisis, you act while others freeze. This decisiveness becomes your reputation. Your reputation builds trust. Trust creates opportunities. Opportunities generate success. Success compounds.

Watch how it cascades:

Discipline in training → You show up when you don't feel like it. You push through pain. You master fundamentals through repetition.

Physical transformation → Your body changes. You move differently. You carry yourself with purpose. Others notice.

Confidence emerges → Not arrogance—quiet certainty. You've tested yourself under pressure. You know what you're capable of.

Presence commands respect → People respond to confidence. They defer to it. They want to be around it. Doors open.

Trust is earned → You demonstrate discipline. You show up. You follow through. People learn they can count on you.

Opportunities multiply → When people trust you, they bring you opportunities. The job offer. The partnership. The introduction to someone influential.

Success builds on success → Each win makes the next one easier. Your network expands. Your skills deepen. Your confidence grows. The compound effect accelerates.

Most people understand success as a destination. Something you arrive at through the right combination of ambition, opportunity, and timing. They're waiting for the conditions to be right. They're waiting for the break that changes the trajectory.

They'll wait a long time.

What martial training delivers — not through philosophy but through direct physical experience, Monday after Monday, year after year — is that success is *not a destination*. It's a direction. And the direction compounds.

It starts somewhere completely unglamorous.

You show up to train when you don't feel like it. You just show up because you said you would and that still means something to you. You do the fundamental drills that you've done hundreds of times without visible improvement and you do them again. You absorb a hard session, sleep on it, wake up sore, and return.

Nobody is watching. Nothing has changed yet. This is the part that separates the people who transform from the people who only tried for a while.

Then the body changes. Not all at once — gradually, then suddenly, the way most real things shift. You move differently. The posture changes first, the way you occupy space. People who haven't seen you in six months say something. People who see you every day can't quite name it but they feel it. You've stopped apologizing for being in the room and you didn't even notice when that stopped.

The confidence that arrives from physical transformation is a different animal from the confidence people perform in boardrooms and networking events. That kind is borrowed — it depends on circumstances remaining favorable. This kind is structural. You've been to your edge and you know where it is. You've been tested under conditions that were uncomfortable and you know how you respond. Nobody can give you that knowledge and nobody can take it away.

Quiet certainty is the phrase. Not arrogance — arrogance is compensation. This is simply a man or woman who has done the work and carries the knowledge of it without needing to announce it.

And here's where it gets interesting.

That quality is legible to other people in ways they often can't articulate. Presence that comes from genuine capability reads differently than presence that comes from performance. People respond to it. They defer to it in moments of uncertainty. They want proximity to it. The person who remains composed when the situation deteriorates — who acts with clarity while others are still processing whether to panic — that person becomes the one the room turns toward.

That attention, sustained over time, becomes trust. And trust is the actual currency. Not credentials. Not connections. Not the right school or the right title. The simple, earned, demonstrated fact that when you say you'll do something, it happens. When the situation demands someone who won't fold, you are that person and the people around you have watched you prove it enough times that they no longer question it.

What trust generates — quietly, without announcement — is access.

The conversation that leads to the opportunity. The introduction to the person who changes the trajectory. The partnership offered to you specifically because someone who could have chosen anyone decided they wanted the person they could count on. These things don't arrive as rewards. They arrive as logical conclusions. The world routes opportunity toward reliability the way water finds the path of least resistance — not randomly, not fairly, but consistently.

And then the compounding begins in earnest.

Each success recalibrates your sense of what's possible. Your network deepens because the people you attract at one level of performance are different from the people you attracted before. Your skills sharpen because you're now operating in environments that demand more. Your confidence isn't performing anymore — it's just accurate. You know what you can do because you've watched yourself do it, repeatedly, under pressure, when it mattered.

This is what nobody tells you is inside the training.

They tell you about the fitness. The self-defense. The discipline. All true, all real, all valuable. But underneath all of it, quietly accumulating across the years, is a person being rebuilt at the foundation — someone whose relationship with difficulty, with discomfort, with the gap between where they are and where they intend to be, has fundamentally changed.

This can be exponential. Like interest compounding in an account, each addition to your capabilities generates returns that themselves generate more returns. The black belt who trained for ten years doesn't just have ten years of experience—they have ten years of compounding development where each year's growth built on the years prior.

Train Harder Than Life

If the hard road is the way to victory, make all training as hard as possible. The harder training is, the easier life will seem. This is the positive feedback cascade. Each brutal training session cuts another facet into your diamond—precise, deliberate, transformative. When you train beyond what's necessary, when you prepare for worst-case scenarios, when you push yourself to the absolute limit in practice, you're not just building strength or skill. You're adding facets that catch light from every angle. The actual challenges life throws at you become manageable by comparison because you've already honed yourself against worse. The more difficult the cut, the more brilliant the surface. The more you polish under pressure, the more you shine when it matters.

Many high-level athletes go on to become successful business owners. They know getting up early and staying late only keeps you in the game. What you need is an understanding of the competition and how to organize, plan, and execute a strategy to win. The tools used to assist your progress as a martial artist—discipline, strategy, relentless refinement—are the same that can be applied to all parts of your life.

Building Your Army

Here's another compounding effect: relationships. The more you give, the more you receive—but not immediately. You invest in people. You help them advance. You support their growth. Over time, these investments compound.

Popular people are that way because they're comfortable in social interactions, thinking and acting quickly to new information and unexpected challenges. They've had experience under pressure and stepped up when the heat was on. They have confidence in themselves. They've proven themselves. They've also built relationships. They've invested in people. They've built their army one person at a time.

When you give of yourself—your body in training, your time in helping others develop—they return the favor. Maybe not right away, but your efforts don't go unnoticed. People you don't even know are paying attention and will recognize your contributions. Put in enough effort over enough time, and you'll have friends and allies who will support and lift you far above where you could have reached alone.

This is the greatest level of wealth: the love, respect, and support of those around you. Material wealth also comes with opportunities from those who respect you and want to see you advance. Many benefits spin off from building community and supporting others.

My Two Rules for Happiness and Success

Happiness is having fun doing what you want to do, all the time. Here's how:

RULE #1: Control your time.

Control your time means only doing what's important to you and your goals. Owning your time allows you to achieve goals quickly. As you achieve goals quickly, you'll feel encouraged at the pace of improvement and have more time to get further.

Life is a series of opportunities you must seize, because they may only come once. You'll be 23 once, and the next thing you're 30. Make the most of that age too, because you're 40 before you know it. And so on. Carpe diem. Seize the day.

Ask yourself these questions every day:

1. **What do you want to do in your life right now?** Learn piano, fly a plane, dance, or draw? Shoot guns or rock climb? Build a house or learn to knit? Write a book about dragons and princesses or paint a masterpiece? Answer honestly and then do it.
2. **Where do you want to go in the future?** Live in the city or on a farm, maybe the deep wilderness? Live with other people or just pets? Want a deep loving relationship? Or travel around and see the sights solo? Your destination matters.
3. **What people do you want around you now and in the future?** You become the average of the people you spend time with. If you have someone in your life with a character trait you have a problem with and don't want to adopt, help them fix it quick or

decide if you want to take on a little of that flaw.

4. **How can you make money doing something you like right now?** What are your natural skills? Can you teach something? Making money proves you have a commercially viable skill. Society wants what you're offering and will give up some of their energy and money to do it with you. That's a privilege and a vouch that you're doing something of measurable value.

After asking and answering these questions every day for ten years, you'll be ten years further down the road of a successful life. A meaningful, joyful, painful, learning, and growing experience that you can share with others and help them be successful too.

RULE #2: Make everything fun.

My favorite: Make everything fun. The mind trick is to start every new task and say, this will be fun! Others will appreciate your grit and determination and respect you for doing it with a great attitude. Do it enough times, and respect will grow and you'll toughen your character. If you control your time, then you are doing something that serves your purpose anyway. So even if it sucks, you need to do it, and it is for your ultimate benefit, so best enjoy what you can out of making your life better.

That's it. Two rules. Do them every day and you'll find happiness and success fast.

The Compounding Continues

Every morning is a new opportunity to start fresh. Your past does not define you. If you follow the two rules and start finding success—more money, more problems, right? You now need systems to ensure you keep what you've earned. The key to managing success: A. Don't get lost in it. B. Don't take it for granted. C. Maintain and grow.

To compound your successes, add more to the mix. More experiences, more knowledge, more humility, more love, more respect, more trust, more connection to your existence. By constantly building on what we have, the minor setbacks life throws at us are quickly forgotten.

People are your most valuable resource. If you've surrounded yourself with high-quality people, help them advance on their path. Bring them with you for the ride. Friends of high quality are rare and need cultivation and encouragement.

Maximum effort equals maximum effect. Self-development leads to mind, body, and spirit in harmony, in balance, and equals better whole-of-life performance. A high-performing individual is accepted into the peer group they desire based on positive outcomes and self-control that shines when goals are made and met at higher than average rates. The rich and powerful want successful people around themselves.

The Path of Success

Here's what I'm telling you: if you get the trinity trained right— your mind, body and spirit (scholar, lover, warrior)—if you nurture your relationships, apply discipline to your goals, and follow the road-map we have examined, you will achieve whatever level of wealth and success you want. Not might. Will. It's all achievable.

When you train your body to peak capability, your mind to clarity, and your spirit to flow with the Tao, you can see the results in the mirror. You feel it in your health. People sense it before you speak. They're drawn to it without understanding why. This is the magnetism of the complete warrior—not arrogance, not aggression, but quiet power combined with genuine respect for yourself and others.

When you're strong but don't need to prove it, when you're capable of violence but choose peace, when you respect yourself deeply and therefore extend that respect outward—opportunities open. Allies materialize. Conflicts dissolve before they escalate. People want your energy around them. They want your hard work, your can-do attitude, your disciplined approach to problems. They want to be near someone who has their shit together.

This is the warrior's competitive advantage in life, not just in combat. The refined martial artist leads with these attractive energies—discipline, respect, calm power, genuine confidence—and follows up with predictable excellent results. Success breeds success. Respect compounds. Wealth in all its forms accumulates.

True success is personal pride rooted in humility. Riches based in respect. Accomplishments borne of love for yourself and others. A clear mind and conscience. No guilt of the past and no fear of the future. The scholar, the lover, and the warrior operating simultaneously in perfect balance—thinking clearly, loving deeply, and acting decisively in the same breath.

This is what the martial path builds. Not just fighting ability. Complete human capability.

The Dalai Lama warned: "Man sacrifices his health to make money, then sacrifices money to recoup his health. He is so anxious about the future that he is not in the present. He lives as if he will never die, then dies having never really lived."

Don't be that person. You know better now. Bring yourself into the present and operate from there.

You've been given the tools: the OODA loop, time management, the emergency button, Zen flow, the Tao, visualization, the diamond metaphor, the three archetypes, fear management, spiritual activation, physical training methods. You understand that discipline transfers, that training creates wealth in all forms, that maximum effort equals maximum effect.

Now comes the only part that matters: doing it.

This is the warrior's path to success. Not because fighting makes you successful, but because the discipline, the dedication, the relentless pursuit of excellence, the ability to make decisions under pressure, the willingness to face your fears, the commitment to never quit—these qualities transfer to everything you do.

Maintaining steady improvement and dedication to mastering yourself physically, mentally, and spiritually is a task never completed. Know that every incremental advancement produces exponential returns. Your accomplishments multiply. Respect from yourself and others inevitably follows. Opportunities appear. Allies emerge. Success becomes your default trajectory.

You already possess everything you need. The elements for success are inside you, waiting to be refined. The rough diamond is already there—you are both the stone and the master craftsman.

Enter the martial way. The best time to start was yesterday. The next best time is now.

Start now, join me in training and growing rich.

"Success is the result of preparation, hard work, and learning from failure."—Chuck Norris, 1988

Thank you for reading this book, your 30 second review on Amazon would be very meaningful for my journey;

https://www.amazon.com/review/create-review?&asin=B0G4NFFWX8

Email: WhoTrainsWins@proton.me

Code: BLACKBELT90 - whotrainswins.com

Appendix

Eight Virtues of Bushido;
1. Justice
2. Courage
3. Benevolence
4. Respect
5. Sincerity
6. Honor
7. Loyalty
8. Self Control

21 Tenets of Miyamoto Musashi;
1. Accept everything just the way it is.
2. Do not seek pleasure for its own sake.
3. Do not, under any circumstances, depend on a partial feeling.
4. Think lightly of yourself and deeply of the world.
5. Be detached from desire your whole life long.
6. Do not regret what you have done.
7. Never be jealous.
8. Never let yourself be saddened by a separation.
9. Resentment and complaint are not appropriate for oneself nor others.
10. Do not let yourself be guided by lust or love.
11. In all things have no preferences.
12. Be indifferent to where you live.
13. Do not pursue the taste of good food.
14. Do not hold on to possessions no longer needed.
15. Do not act following customary beliefs.
16. Do not collect or practice with weapons beyond what is useful.

17. Do not fear death.

18. Do not seek to possess either goods or fiefs for your old age.

19. Respect the gods without counting on their help.

20. You may abandon your own body but you must preserve your honor.

21. Never stray from the Way.

Taoist Training Mantra;

Down, Up, Same Time
In, Out, Same Breath
Left, Right, Same Side
Hand, Foot, Same Body
Hand, Foot, Same Intent
Right, Left, Same Speed
Out, In, Same Ki
Up, Down, Same Time

Shaolin's 7 Principles;

- **Never Give Up** – If your heart is strong, you can accomplish anything. Once you have decided on your Shaolin goal, cut off any road of retreat. Advance like an arrow from a bow. Burn your boats. Give yourself no choice.

- **Always Practice** – Shaolin Martial Arts is like boiling water, if you do not keep the flame high with continued training, your skill turns tepid. Standing, sleeping, awake or asleep, the Shaolin Warrior always practices. Never separate yourself from the way of the warrior.

- **Integrate Yin And Yang** – You are not learning techniques, you are learning nature. The integration of Yin and Yang training is the essence of Shaolin. Every time you do your Shaolin Workout the positive energy of heaven and earth is inhaled.

- **Turn Yourself Into Zero** – When we enter the temple, we prostrate 3 times, this is a symbol of letting go of our body, speech and mind. Let go and entrust everything that comes up in your life – anxiety, illness, stress – to your Shaolin Practice.

- **Nurture Your Body** – Your body is a treasured gift from heaven and earth. Using medicine is a last resort. If you take care of yourself, eat well, do Shaolin Qigong, you will not become ill. Don't neglect your bodies basic health

- **Apply Great Effort** – If you put a lot of effort into your Shaolin Martial Arts and don't become very skilful at it, you have still excelled yourself. Because whether you're good or bad at your training, the result is the same: it's one of the most positive things you can do for your mind and body

- **Cut Off Desire** – People's minds get tangled up in objects and this fragments their energy and hinders their practice. Only have what you really need rather than what you really want. Happiness come from our internal world, not from the external.

(Courtesy – Shifu Yan Lei)

Five Tenets of Tae Kwon Do:

1. **Courtesy** (Ye'Ue):

Always be kind and humble to others to make them comfortable and pleased with you.

2. **Integrity** (JungJik):

Always be honest and have a strong sense of right and wrong. The degree of wrong does not matter; wrong is wrong.

3. **Perseverance** (In Nae):

Always be patient and diligent in achieving your goals. Success comes to only those who persevere.

4. **Self Control** (GuekKee):

Always be in control of your emotions and your surroundings. True respect comes only from self-control.

5. **Indomitable Spirit** (BaekJuhlBoolGool):

Whenever confronted with injustice, always deal with the situation without fear of outcome or reprisal.

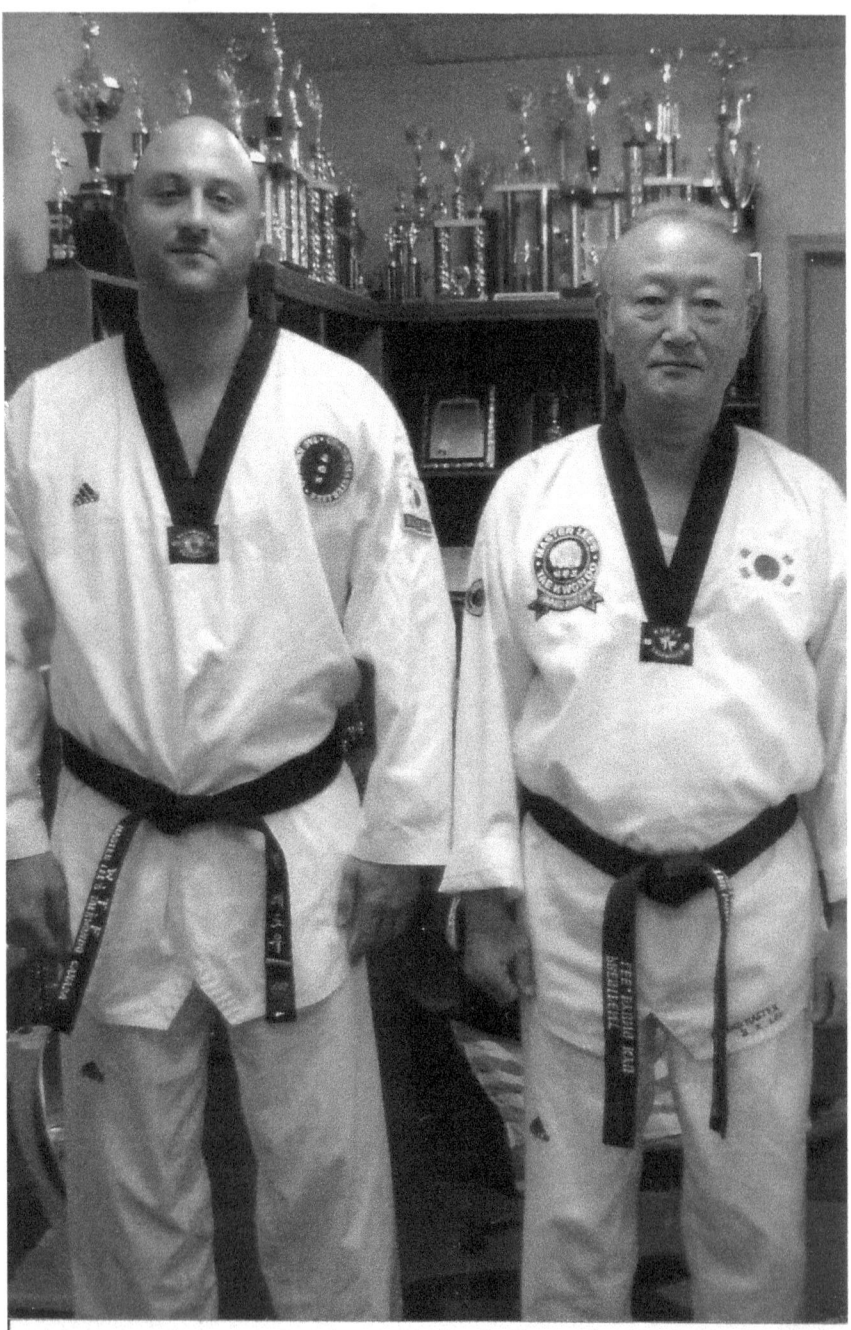

Acknowledgments

DEDICATION;

To my true love and whose respect powers my soul, Erika Turnbull. You mean more to me than you will ever know. You are an amazing human – par excellence.

FRIENDS;

Wesley – more plates, more dates
Andrew – work ethic
Gordon – fastest OODA
Kevin – warrior poet
Richard – calm under fire
Hiroyuki – respect
Jeff – honor
My Czech Shepherds – Draco and Atos – always ready

INSTRUCTORS & MENTORS – giants on whose shoulders I stand;

Kwanjang Byung Kyu Lee — legacy and wisdom (masterlee.ca)

Sabonim Song Young Lee – warrior on the mountain (Master Lees TKD, Abbotsford BC)

Sifu John Fowler – value of meditation (Chilliwack Kung-fu/Muay Thai)

Master Trainer Tony Nikl – train the alpha beast (CANCZECHDOGS.com)

Coach Kultar Gill — dedication (mambamma.com/)

Coach Darren Macdonald — the humble warrior (smoothcomp.com/en/profile/1015649)

Coach Bas Rutten — difficult training for easy fights (basrutteninstructionals.com/)

Mestre Alberto Crane — bullies are great motivators (Legacybjj.com)

Dr. Manjit Gosel — Kaizen Medical — health & zen (kaizenmed.com/)

Dr. Masaaki Hatsumi Soke — venerable origin spark (bujinkan.com/)

Guro Dan Inosanto — learning never ends (Inosanto Academy of Martial Arts)

Sheriff James Yeager — always prepared for the fight (tacticalresponse.com/)

Instructor Craig Douglas – rules change, adapt (shivworks.com/)

Bibliography

Berg, Eric. 2017. The Seven Principles of Fat Burning. KB Publishers.

Blumenstein, Boris et al. 2002. Brain and Body in Sport and Exercise. John Wiley and Sons Ltd.

Chuen, Lam Kam. 1997. The Way of Energy: Chinese Art of Internal Strength. Simon and Schuster.

Canney, James C. 2008. Health and Fitness in the Martial Arts. McFarland & Company.

de Becker, Gavin. 1997. The Gift of Fear: Survival Signals That Protect Us from Violence. Little, Brown and Company.

Deshimaru, Taisen. 1982. The Zen Way to the Martial Arts. Translated by Nancy Amphoux. E.P. Dutton.

Draeger, Donn F. and Smith, Robert W. 1980. Comprehensive Asian Martial Fighting Arts. Kodansha Int. Ltd.

Emoto, Masaru. 2004. The Hidden Messages in Water. Beyond Words Publishing.

Feng, Gia–Fu, and English, Jane. 1972. Lao Tsu –Tao Te Ching. Random House Publishing.

Goleman, Daniel. 1995. Emotional Intelligence: Why It Can Matter More Than IQ. Bantam Books.

Griffith, Samuel B. 1963. Sun Tzu The Art of War. Oxford University Press

Grossman, David, Lt. Col. 2004. On Combat. Warrior Science Publications.

Harwood–Gross, A., et al. 2021. The Effect of Martial Arts Training on Cognitive and Psychological Functions in At–Risk Youths. *Frontiers in Pediatrics*, 9.

Howe, Paul R. 2005. Leadership and Training for the Fight from a former Special Operations Soldier. Authorhouse Publishing.

Kim, Richard. 1982. The Classical Man. Ohara Publications.

Lakes, K. D., and W. T. Hoyt. 2004. Promoting self–regulation through school–based martial arts training. Applied Developmental Psychology 25(3).

Lee, Bruce. 1975. Tao of Jeet Kune Do. Ohara Publications.

Musashi, Miyamoto. 1974. The Book of Five Rings. Translated by Victor Harris. Overlook Press.

O'Neill, Barbara. 2012. Self Heal by Design: The Role of Micro-Organisms for Health. Self-published.

Ranganathan, V. K., Siemionow, V., Liu, J. Z., Sahgal, V., & Yue, G. H. (2004). From mental power to muscle power—gaining strength by using the mind. *Neuropsychologia*, 42(7), 944–956.

Rosenbaum, Michael. 1998. Kata and the Transmission of Knowledge in Traditional Martial Arts. YMAA Publication Center.

Selby, John. 2003. Seven Masters, One Path: Meditation Secrets from the World's Greatest Teachers. HarperOne.

Siddle, Bruce K. 1995. Sharpening the Warriors Edge. The Psychology & Science of Training. PPCT Research Publications.

Suarez, Gabe. 2003. The Combative Perspective; The Thinking Man's Guide to Self-Defense. Paladin Press.

Tabata, Kazumi. 2003. Secret Tactics: Lessons from the Great Masters of the Martial Arts. Tuttle Publishing.

Wise, Jeff. 2009. Extreme Fear: The Science of your Mind in Danger. St. Martins Press.

About The Author; Certifications and Courses (Abbreviated)

Aim Fast Hit Fast – 2008
ASIS International Member – 2019
BCSC; Security Consultant Designation – 2018
BJJ – 2002
Boxing – 2016
Caliber 3 IDF Intro 3 gun – 2019
Canadian BC Security Worker Licence – 2017
Canadian Open TKD Championships 1998
Canadian Provincials TKD – 1997
CJ Lawrence / Secret Service (Rt) – Risk Assessment Tools – 2018
CPIRC – Investigations Officer Certificate – 2018
CTOMS – Officer down Survival Course – 2020
DMSS Convoy Sec. & Mounted Ops – 2005
Douglas College New West – Investigations
FireArms Academy ECQC – 2007
Freddie Spencer's Driving School – 2003
Grandmaster Lee's Open 3rd – 1997
Greenline Tactical – Low light – 2005
Greenline Tactical – DMR/SPR – 2005
Innosanto Academy of Martial Arts – Instructor skills – 2014
IPSC Competitors Black Badge – 2004
J.DeGroot – High Risk Contractor ;ASSET & VIP Protection – 2017
J.Degroot – Compound and Perimeter Security – 2018
Kendo – 1999
Kung Fu Shaolin – 1986
LMS Defense Pistol – 2008
LMS Defense Carbine 2 – 2008
Norske Tac AirCraft Protection Series I, II, III – 2003
PIABC – Professional Investigator Development Seminar – 2019
Presidential Cup TKD Championship 2nd – 1999
Private Pilots Licence Fixed/Night/Mountain – 2010
Private Pilots Licence Float – 2011
PSTN Investigations Certificate – 2016
Rhodes Solutions – Combat First Aid – 2017
ShivWorks – Knife Fighting & Defense – 2008
ShivWorks – Sim force on force/Int scenarios – 2007
Shotokan Karate – 2003
SigArms Academy Pistol Skills – 2004
SimTactical Force on Force CQB – 2005
St John Ambulance CPR C w AED (recert) – 2011
St John Ambulance Intermediate First aid – 2004

St John Ambulance Standard First Aid – 2011
STOAS – Professional Surveillance Package – 2017
Tactical Response Advanced Fighting Pistol – 2007
Tactical Response Advanced Fighting Rifle – 2007
Tactical Response Fighting Pistol – 2006
Tactical Response Fighting Rifle – 2006
TKD Official Judges Certification – 1998
Toddington Inter. Investigations – 2017
Toddington Inter. Intelligence Analysis – 2019
Toddington Inter. OSINT Certification – 2017
UBC– Criminology & Investigations
UFV – Law & Criminology 2009–2012
UFV – Psychology & Sociology 2010–2011
Veritac Solutions Dismounted Small Teams Operations – 2017
Veritac Solutions Multi Weapon Operations – 2017
VS Training & Combat Medical/TCCC – 2012
W.Place Inv. Interviews & Techniques – 2017
W.Place Training Institute – Investigations + 4 Certifications – 2017
WTF TKD Kukkiwon Black Belt Certification – 2009
X Tactical – Extreme Weather Survival – 2008

www.ingramcontent.com/pod-product-compliance
Lightning Source LLC
Chambersburg PA
CBHW060455090426
42735CB00011B/1993